"*Yoga Therapy as a Creative Response to Pain* is a provocative, yet humorous, book that will likely shake, stir, and then ultimately expand your notion of yoga therapy, in ways that will deeply reward you both professionally and personally... And maybe even move you a little further towards eudaimonia."

—*from the Foreword by John Kepner, MA, MBA C-IAYT, Executive Director of the International Association of Yoga Therapists*

"Integrating pain science, yoga, and creativity, Taylor masterfully introduces a new paradigm for patient care. A must-read for all healthcare professionals seeking a novel and effective approach for the treatment of chronic pain."

—*Dr. Lori Rubenstein Fazzio, DPT, PT, MAppSc, C-IAYT, Loyola Marymount University Yoga Studies Faculty, Clinical Director of Yoga Therapy Rx, and CEO of Mosaic Physical Therapy of related interest*

Yoga for a Happy Back
A Teacher's Guide to Spinal Health
through Yoga Therapy
Rachel Krentzman, PT, E-RYT
Foreword by Aadil Palkhivala
ISBN 978 1 84819 271 3
eISBN 978 0 85701 253 1

Yoga Therapy for Parkinson's Disease
and Multiple Sclerosis
Jean Danford
ISBN 978 1 84819 299 7
eISBN 978 0 85701 249 4

Principles and Themes in Yoga Therapy
An Introduction to Integrative Mind/
Body Yoga Therapeutics
James Foulkes
Foreword by Mikhail Kogan, MD
Illustrated by Simon Barkworth
ISBN 978 1 84819 248 5
eISBN 978 0 85701 194 7

Yoga Teaching Handbook
A Practical Guide for Yoga Teachers and Trainees
Edited by Sian O'Neill
ISBN 978 1 84819 355 0
eISBN 978 0 85701 313 2

Scoliosis, Yoga Therapy, and the Art of Letting Go
Rachel Krentzman, PT, E-RYT
Foreword by Matthew J. Taylor PT, PhD
ISBN 978 1 84819 272 0
eISBN 978 0 85701 243 2

YOGA THERAPY *as a* Creative Response to Pain

Matthew J. Taylor

Foreword by John Kepner

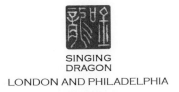

SINGING
DRAGON
LONDON AND PHILADELPHIA

First published in 2018
by Singing Dragon
an imprint of Jessica Kingsley Publishers
73 Collier Street
London N1 9BE, UK
and
400 Market Street, Suite 400
Philadelphia, PA 19106, USA

www.singingdragon.com

Library of Congress Cataloging in Publication Data
A CIP catalog record for this book is available from the Library of Congress

British Library Cataloguing in Publication Data
A CIP catalogue record for this book is available from the British Library

ISBN 978 1 84819 356 7
eISBN 978 0 85701 315 6

Printed and bound in Great Britain

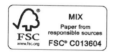

Dedication

To my colleagues worldwide who "see" the
better future we are creating. May we conspire to
co-create a future that transforms our suffering and
reflects the inherent dignity of being human.

Contents

Foreword

Yoga Therapy as a Creative Response to Pain is a provocative, yet humorous, book that will likely shake, stir, and then ultimately expand your notion of yoga therapy, in ways that will deeply reward you both professionally and personally… And maybe even move you a little further towards *eudaimonia*.

There is an urgent need to address chronic pain in our society. Chronic pain is the most prevalent, costly, and disabling health condition in the US. Matthew Taylor, PT, PhD, C-IAYT, and a former President of the Board of the International Association of Yoga Therapists (IAYT) is the yoga therapy representative to the Integrative Healthcare Policy Consortium on Chronic Pain and Opioid Abuse, but his book will *not* provide typical yogic technological answers for yoga therapists and others working in this area. What it *will* provide is a stream of self-deprecating stories, amusingly presented provocative questions, multiple suggestions within a learned yet pragmatic philosophical framework, an incredible set of references, and last, but not least, a large collection of recommended "practices." The integrated sum provides an informed choice for yoga professionals: a) to slog through the draining work of addressing the pain of their clients (and themselves) *or* b) to approach their work (with his brilliant guidance) "with the intention of viewing this work as a potential opportunity for discovery and the innate 'fun' of satisfying human curiosity through discovery." For many, this may be both revolutionary and immensely personally satisfying.

Matt, despite his many credentials, is really a *karma* yogi at heart. Early in my time with IAYT, in the 90s, physical therapists would call me, curious about yoga therapy and how that might augment their PT practice. I would say, "Talk to Matt Taylor," and almost inevitably they would say, "I know him, he helped me with this, or reviewed my book, or spoke at my studio, etc., etc." For Matt is a selfless spirit, always generously helping others, knowing that through service it will come back to support him and, in turn, enable him to serve more. That same spirit of generosity is woven throughout the book for you.

Another time he and I did a workshop together. I gave a learned lecture, so I thought; but when his turn came, he had the audience immediately break into small groups, to ask their own questions and share their own answers with their peers, knowing that the process of shared collaborative discovery is the best discovery. That idea, of collaborative learning, is also the foundation of IAYT's Common Interest Community sessions that Matt founded and that we have offered at the start of our conferences for many years—bringing people together, right at the start of a big conference, to share their successes (and sometimes failures). These then often initiated collaborative learning efforts that persisted throughout the rest of the conference and years afterwards. And it is this powerful, shared collaborative approach with which *Yoga Therapy as a Creative Response to Pain* calls the reader to "be with" vs. "to do to" the client.

So, in sum, this book brings together Matt's humbling experience with his own excruciating pain and then years of personal yoga study, remarkable scholarship, generous service orientation, and his long experience with collaborative learning to guide you through asking your own questions and coming up with your own (always tentative) answers. From this truly substantive foundation, you can make your own way so you can ultimately serve your clients, and yourself, in a more effective and satisfying way.

John Kepner, MA, MBA, C-IAYT
Executive Director, International Association of Yoga Therapists

Acknowledgments

The premise of this book is that creativity never happens in isolation. My trying to draft this acknowledgment section underscores the depth and accuracy of that premise.

This book began because my dear friend Lori Rubenstein-Fazzio, DPT, PT, MAppSc, C-IAYT was too over-committed to accept the book offer from Singing Dragon. Lori referred the wonderful Claire Wilson of Singing Dragon to me, and the rest, as they say, is history. Much gratitude to each of you for enabling this "possible."

When I reflect on my wisdom teachers, I first think of my parents, Mary and Jerry Taylor. Without their foundational training and modeling, this book would never happen. I want to acknowledge my direct teachers, many of whom are no longer living, but each continues to guide me. My thanks go to my first boss and mentor, Fred Jesse, PT, Col. (Ret); Fr. Mike Librandi for teaching me to ask questions of authority; Dick Alexander, JD, mentor who taught me to think deeply; Don Gereau, master of generating options/new possibles; Ray Collins, my father in-law, for his salt and light; Fr. Matthew Fox, for his scholarship and insights; Brian Swimme, PhD, for his Universe story; Alfonso Montuori, PhD, my dissertation chair and friend, for his care and tending my progression into complexity; Joseph LePage,

MA, Larry Payne, PhD, and Richard Miller, PhD, for sharing their yoga and reintroducing me to myself; Charlie Trull, PhD, my lilac brother who never lets me down; Michael Lee, MA, mate from Down Under, wise man, and he who asks the obvious, but important, questions; and Staffan Elgelid, PT, PhD, GCFP, C-IAYT, you know you are to blame, right? The one that brings the Viking out in me.

My immediate family forms my foundation. My three amazing children: Emily, Adam, and Anthony provide the flame that inspires me to make a meaningful contribution to creating a best future for them and their loved ones. Ultimately though, my knowing wisdom is because of the love of my life for over 40 years now, Jennifer. She is my Sophia and, by my good fortune, she has stuck with me to show me that I am too. I'm a lucky guy.

Preface

Two and half sheets of wallboard, 26 nails per sheet, and one big, lazy fat fly touring the ceiling. That was my view for one week in a cabin in northern Minnesota. My persistent back pain had been building for over a decade and finally brought me down after a 12-hour drive in the family Suburban. The highly respected and successful back pain specialist, the back-fixer, needed fixing. The iconic week in the woods became a week flat on my back, barely able to get to the bathroom. Embarrassing, frustrating, humbling, scary, depressing, and not a little anger provoking. Knowing enough to be alarmed, knowing too much for my own good, and finding all my wisdom for eliminating back pain was of no value. Little did I realize that this low point in my life was also a doorway that would lead to a very different me 22 years later.

. . .

We will return to the northern woods of Minnesota in each chapter of the book to see what happened to this fit, 37-year-old owner of a sports medicine rehabilitation clinic and gym, father of three, sole bread-winner, and all-around good community guy from small town middle America. What I can tell you now, though, is he'd never have imagined today he'd be sitting in Arizona, outside in the sun on a winter afternoon, writing a book about wisdom, pain, yoga therapy, and creativity: Surprise! ... I didn't see this coming.

But what I really want to know is, what would you as a yoga professional (defined as either teacher or therapist for the remainder of the book), what would you have done for me if I was your student?

What stories would you have told me? What kind of history would you have asked of me? What would you tell me you could do for me given my circumstance? How would you keep me from surgery? Would I leave hopeful or discouraged? Would I know "me" better because of my time with you? Would I be any wiser? More creative? Emboldened? In less pain? Empowered with a strategy for living with my pain? Would you have presumed to know what I needed? Were you recently at the "Yoga for Back Pain" workshop and now had just the right sequence for my symptoms? How would you deal with a conventional medical expert in back pain as a student? Would you understand what meaning my pain and suffering had for me? For you? I know, a great deal of questions from a guy that is considered to be an expert, right?

And that is my point. Thirty-six years of practice, endless degrees, and training, and I still have far more questions than answers. I am now quite sure that having more questions than answers is the way this is all going to play out in my lifetime, too. Rats, more questions than answers. And that's OK, unless you picked up this book hoping to get all the answers. But hold on, allow me to ask you a couple of questions first and see if we can't find something very important to explore together, shall we?

Stop and consider: With the information boom, fancy MRI studies, and so many books, seminars, and potions for eliminating pain, why does pain become a bigger problem every year? Not just a little bigger, but by multiples. The costs in terms of suffering, lost opportunity, and wrecked human relationships aren't even included in the statistics. Are we missing something, perhaps? Are we even possibly doing something to make matters worse? Yes, even we well-intentioned yoga professionals? Maybe the pain is supposed to be leading us somewhere rather than just be something to overcome or "win the war" with? What if, instead of following those pervasive patterns of our society, we (the human species this time) were to create something beyond our imaginations that celebrated and fostered behavior that reflected that yoga–Unity thing about all of us being connected? How would you and I need to change? Would you be willing to change? Could you surrender your current understanding of who you are and why you teach yoga philosophy and technologies? I know I'm getting personal here, but I'm also asking that of myself as I write. In the autumn of 2017 as we survey the landscape of our planet, is there not a sense of some urgency for change that exceeds what you and I have previously experienced in our lifetime?

I believe this need for change of course includes the alleviation and prevention of suffering, as we're charged in Patanjali's Yoga Sutra II.16: *Heyam duhkham anagatam*: Prevent the suffering that is yet to come. Pain as you know is part of that suffering, but not the same thing. Yoga therapy offers a creative response to the suffering we see, but not if it's taught from the common prescriptive Western model alone. We teach that we are all connected, and that means you and I are both responsible for the state of our world, *and* have the power to transform it. I believe we are up to the task of transforming suffering and our world. Join me, won't you, in the pages ahead to question, deconstruct, reflect, and then act, as a creative response to the suffering in ourselves, our communities, and the world.

Introduction

Disclaimer: The opinions expressed in this book are mine. Some will prove accurate, some not so much. Unfortunately, I can't tell you which is which. If I do my job correctly, there will be several sacrilegious yoga perspectives that may offend some in the yoga community. There will also be a few heretical statements that will offend some of my conventional healthcare peers. No offense intended, but the fact that someone will be offended is certainly expected. And it is my "yoga" to write as authentically as I can and not edit to avoid disturbing themes. I would guess I'm not the only one that grew up in that "don't rock the boat" familial culture. Besides who needs one more solemn, serious yoga book you probably didn't finish that is sitting on your shelves? I am certainly no sage or avatar, but I am deeply compelled to offer my limited understanding in our crazy current life context. This will be fun...especially if I don't take myself too seriously. You are invited to do the same: that is, not to take me, or yourself, too seriously.

Please allow me to get a few contentious, uncomfortable ideas out of the way so we can get to the fun stuff:

1. Your and my understanding of yoga and how we teach is deeply tainted by our cultural perspectives leading to a good deal of unintended avidyâ and asmitâ as a source of suffering.

2. What we know about pain is at best incomplete, and much of it won't be true in five years no matter how complete our understanding is right now.

3. There will be no algorithms, formulas, or recipes; this is not a technician's step by step guide. We are all professionals here, not technicians following a checklist.

4. What we understand and believe about creativity is both incomplete and almost certainly incongruent with our current yoga understanding and practice.

5. Yoga therapy is emerging and evolving. There is no fixed "right way" to "do" yoga therapy. Sorry.

6. Same goes for wisdom teachings in general. We build on the traditions, but the challenging teachings are also reinterpreted in light of constant change, and therefore in need of fresh perspective. "Now is now." Not sure who said that, but it places an important responsibility on each one of us: now.

With that out of the way, allow me share just a few insights about me, the author. To start, as I said in the Preface, I'm loaded with questions and I know that I don't know all the answers. Second, I tend to hide behind big words and complicated thoughts, so I will ~~endeavor~~ try to write ~~lucidly~~ plainly and ~~ingenuously~~ simply. Third, I really am a pretty nice guy, but I feel an urgency to be more direct and emphatic given the state of things on our planet, so I may come off a bit brusk: but in a nice way. Last, I'm very grateful for your attention, so enough about me and let's get to work.

The foundational activity in this book is paying attention and learning to see, then manage the {SPACE} between a stimulus (S) and your response (R). Here in this book you will find new ways to experience that {SPACE} in first you, then your students. You know that famous quote I'm sure, "Between stimulus and response there is a space. In that space is out power to choose our response. In our response lies our growth and our freedom." You also probably think Victor Frankl said it. Turns out he didn't (Pattakos 2010). Credit Dr. Daniel Siegel (2017) for that fun bit of disruption. Won't this be fun? Anyway, beginning with the completion of the first chapter, you will quite literally begin to see the chaos of modern life differently. As your skills build through each successive chapter, the S{ }R begins to change and with it the quality and choices of your responses will increase. The beauty of the principles is that they work for both you and the organizations/communities to which you belong.

We will explore each of the six contentious ideas listed above. I won't just leave you hanging with those statements. For now, here is a breakdown of the chapters ahead as a roadmap for navigating these fascinating topics. Through this process we will generate many possibilities to explain and understand why there's more pain today despite the increasing number of pain management resources available each year. It will be these new possibilities that will seed the future in hopes of participating in the process of reversing our epidemic of pain.

The Chapters

The flow of the book is constructed to go from what will be most familiar to a yoga professional and then build into each new topic supported by the previous chapters. You can certainly jump around reading those chapters that appear most compelling, but please understand there will be threads between the chapters that will enrich your appreciation of the chapter you might be reading. Here's the lineup ahead and the intended benefits of participating in each chapter:

1. Yoga Isn't What You Think It Is

The first step in creativity is destruction. We begin by deconstructing the common understandings of yoga and I am betting at least a couple of those understandings will be ones you presently hold. Don't worry, though, I won't be offering the "correct" definition either. Thus begins the messiness and play of creating, so it will be safe and fun despite the destruction.

2. Implications from the New Yoga Therapy

It's all well and good to deconstruct our definitions of yoga and yoga therapy, but there should be a good reason to do so. I call this reason the "So what?" factor. If what we teach doesn't have immediate, real world function and practical application, then what was the point? So what? Those points are what we begin to explore in this chapter, laying an adaptable groundwork for the remaining chapters of discovery.

3. Wisdom: That's You

Hey, it's a provocative title, right? Here we explore the wisdom traditions, how our new yoga understanding rests in both the classical and modern teachings. The way those teachings support us as yoga professionals is fascinating and invites so many new possibilities for our work. Like every other chapter, it has to deliver the "So what?" results. How does defining yourself *as* wisdom feel right now? I am not entirely comfortable with the fit myself. I hope you will be more comfortable after soaking in this chapter.

4. A New Understanding of Pain

Let the destruction of creativity mentioned in Chapter 1 continue. This chapter isn't just based on the current pain science literature, but plumbs our understanding of suffering, emergence, and how one teaches from the wisdom of pain. Not coincidentally, you may encounter some uncomfortable cognitive/emotional turbulence traveling through this chapter. What's a pain chapter without a bit of pain? Whether you are starting from scratch in pain theory or are the current expert, I bet we turn at least one old concept around pain on its head for you. Pain can be fun…in a good way.

5. Creativity: You've Got This

We arrive in this chapter with pieces of yoga, wisdom, and pain strewn about. Now what? Yep, break down what you know about creativity in this chapter. There's plenty of nonsense being peddled in the name of creativity these days. We will avoid those misdirections and play with how we can move ahead in creating our best possible futures of decreased pain and suffering. Sorry, I don't have "Five Easy Steps to Creativity" to offer. But you will be cooking up a feast of many new creations after reading this chapter. The weave of the yoga, wisdom, pain, and creativity threads is magnificent to behold.

6. The Fun of Discovery

We laugh and smile far less than we did a decade ago. It's a fact. In this chapter I propose the time for glum solemnity around yoga needs to end. The new-found humility of the previous chapters frees us up to plunge into the deconstructed mess and begin the fun of creating. If we can't have fun, quite frankly I don't believe it's worth doing. Our innate adult curiosity is what theoretically separates us from our primate relatives. This is no time to monkey around. Let's get to the fun "work."

7. Practice Makes Possibles

This big chapter contains all the secrets you didn't know that you needed and will make you glad you read the entire book and paid whatever you paid to own it. Hardly. The chapter is a trove of simple, easy to do, and fun practices. No getting tangled up in figurative or literal knots here. Many will be familiar practices, but nuanced based on the earlier chapters so they become new again. I hope at this point you will also be jotting down your own new practices for yourself and your students. We're creating something that hasn't been before. Together we will have fun easing present suffering and preventing future suffering. The instructions for reaching enlightenment from Patanjali or being invited to play Carnegie Hall are the same, "Practice, practice, practice." Your creating from the wisdom of pain is guaranteed to bring fun and joy into practice.

How to Use This Book

In Chapter 7, "Practice Makes Possibles," the practices are divided roughly by chapter. I opted to put them all together for easier reference as you return for ideas in the future. Having them all in one chapter struck me as easier than paging through the book trying to find the related activities. I included a fair number of citations throughout the book to dive deeper into topics that grab your interest; the full references are at the end of the book. My hope is that you can use this book as a touchstone beyond just a single read. Change is happening at historic high rates and will continue to accelerate. This book is focused on creating relative comfort in this age of uncertainty. As I hinted above, a book of certainty in this age is going to have a short shelf life. This is a book on best practices for being uncertain and should evolve and change each time you return to review sections or seek new possibilities. I think.

Before we start, let's check in with me back in the cabin up north. That poor guy was facing a great deal of uncertainty.

MINNESOTA ADVENTURE

I had no idea what to do next as we pulled away from the cabin in northern Minnesota for the 12-hour drive home. I was carefully tucked in and laid out between the luggage in the back of the Suburban. Sure, I was finally able to walk a bit and sit for a few minutes, but when was this going to "end"? And how was I not going to be like so many of my patients with chronic, debilitating pain? I was, by definition now, a person with chronic, debilitating pain. What I thought I "knew" was no longer certain. This was a different game now. Uncertainty felt very certain. What I had always thought was true wasn't turning out to be Real. I had no way of knowing then that this was my "Introduction" to a process of change and transformation in the deepest sense of those words. Having just read this introduction, possibly I've created some increased uncertainty in what you know? Maybe you were already uncertain and that's why you picked up this book? Or maybe I've made you just angry or upset enough that you'll keep reading just to prove me wrong? All great starting points for our journey ahead from the back of the Suburban. And no, for the parents reading, I didn't get a say on the radio station selection from the three kids just because my back hurt.

1

. . .

Yoga Isn't What You Think It Is

"Relationship is the fundamental truth of this world of appearance."

(Tagore, cited in Ghose 2016, p.98)

MINNESOTA ADVENTURE

Back to the Minnesota cabin… There he lay, Humpty Dumpty, the King of parts, frightened by the prospect he might bump his elbow against the shower wall again generating a lightning bolt of gripping pain across his back and down his leg. So many parts, all nicely organized into a Covey success planner. I had my family life. I had my business life. I had my fitness life. I had my financial life. My spiritual life. My community life. Each with their measurable, dated goals and regularly updated. Holding all those parts tight for safety and "success" like a good, responsible citizen. Constantly throwing myself full force into every new project and goal. Continuing the reverberating pattern of striving for achievement that had made me a high school valedictorian, a "successful" husband, father, and business person all to fulfill some preconception of what it means to be both good and to be secure. I thought. I was doing everything right and now this? Welcome to the universal human cry regarding suffering and the nature of reality, Mr. Taylor. Little did I realize then as the parts expert, do-gooder, and now chronic back pain person, that I was about to learn relationships from a special education high school teacher who taught yoga on the side. He would travel weekly from 20 miles away to my clinic in a town of 3500 people. I thought it was a good business idea. Little did I know.

. . .

Breaking Old Ground

So, you know yoga, right? Are you sure? I'm not so sure. I mean that in a fun, friendly provocative way. Not that I am an authority on classic yoga, by any means. Rather, it is an invitation to let go of what your and my preconceptions of yoga are, then create space for a new understanding to emerge for each of us, including me as the author. So, colleague, consider the following:

Let's play a bit with definitions. Is yoga a thing? Is it a process? Is it static? Is it evolving? If it is evolving, what will it be next? If it isn't evolving, but a static, fixed yoga, which yoga is the correct one? And how might it deal with today's modern challenges? Whose definition is the "correct" one? Why? Which lineage is authentic and why?

I hope you can sense the slippery nature of this line of questioning. Or is defining yoga like the famous US Supreme Court Justice Potter Stewart's definition of obscenity, "I know it when I see it"? Even more slippery is the question of what practices count as a yoga practice? "Classical" asana? Me sitting at this computer aware of my body, breath, thoughts, and emotions while I write? You on your commute with the same qualities of attention? Teaching your child to sense their breath as you both hug after scraping a knee? A multinational corporate board of directors body-sensing after a breathing practice together prior to beginning a strategic planning retreat?

Still sure you know yoga? And we haven't even touched "yoga therapy." Yoga therapy makes yoga look like a set-in-stone, sure thing. Isn't all yoga therapeutic? Aren't we all whole and complete as we are and therefore not in need of a therapeutic intervention? Is it yoga therapy if the guided imagery (bhavana) includes visualizing your genes altering their expression to generate more proteins to build T-cells? What's the Sanskrit term for that? How about going door to door raising community awareness to vote for upgrading the local water safety standards? Talk about an uncomfortable asana, cold calling in your neighborhood for a cause surely must count as asana?

How about if we agree to just be comfortable with a sense of humility and delight in not really knowing what yoga or yoga therapy is? How's that feel? What does that spirit of uncertainty allow to come forward? What are the benefits and limitations of such a state? Does a small (or maybe loud) voice within protest, "But, but..."? It does for me. But behind that voice, sometimes near, and at other times further away, there lies a palpable silence or stillness. Is that yoga? ... Darn, there I go again wanting that certain answer!

Nora Bateson (2017), award-winning filmmaker, writer, and educator on complexity, offers some thoughtful guidance around this discomfort of uncertainty. She acknowledges the "healthy confusion" that comes with the realization that there is more than one way to see something that at first appeared as "certain." She states that the difference between this "confusion," and any "misunderstanding" that we might have had before around what is yoga, is a new humility to learn, and to hold multiple truths at once, especially when they are paradoxical. When we assume certainty, we get misunderstandings; when we see other possibilities, we get to generate the "cognitive dissonance of mutual learning" (2017, p.126) and the healthy confusion that follows. She admonishes that this mutual learning opportunity exists constantly. She states there are no bystanders. So not just defining yoga, but every conversation you have counts. Everywhere. More in Chapter 3 about mutual learning, for now back to yoga definitions.

Following her suggestion, what I would like to propose we try in this chapter is some of the tried and true wisdom of assuming a beginner's mind. We will turn over some of the old, hard-packed soil of yoga stereotypes and myths from the latest post-modern deconstructions. That process of turning over will prep us for the coming chapters about wisdom, pain, and creativity and what might be possible in the future. That future will include not just our personal yoga practices and professional practice, but point to a larger, fresher way of understanding pain and suffering as well as doing the business of yoga. In turning that hard ground over, presumably this different understanding will provoke consideration of the foundational spiritual questions of being human and then how we engage our communities. Which, if I am guessing correctly, will also circle us back around in a repeating pattern of refining our definition of yoga, and on and on, as the kaleidoscope of Reality becomes a small "r" reality of discovery and delight in possible future scenarios.

Before we can do that, as we will learn in Chapter 5 on creativity, there first needs to be destruction and darkness. From the destruction of old learning, we start to see or shine light on new ways of awareness and a tentative new understanding, after which we can move into the fun of discovery. So first, some destruction.

Clodhopper Asana

What's a clodhopper? I'm revealing my Midwestern USA roots. Back in the day of the horse-drawn plow, the clodhopper was the person whose job it was to break up the big clumps, or clods, of hard soil turned over by the single plow blade so that the seeds of new growth could make their way through the soil. Hence, as we break up some hard-packed yoga concepts of the early twenty-first century, we are tilling the ground of our "knowing" for our new growth. Not to worry, you can always return to the hard-packed concepts if you find the clodhopping dissatisfying. (Technically you probably can't, but you can at least try.)

This chapter opened with Tagore's quote about relationship being the fundamental truth of the world of appearance. This early twentieth-century sage with a broad range of interests and expertise saw what modern day science now describes as the foundation for empirical/observable reality. Why I selected relationship as the tip of the plow is because most of modern society, to include me, has been conditioned to see objects and describe reality as objects. This deep conditioning makes it very difficult for us to change our orientation or paradigm. I promise not to flog you with that paradigm word, but it is key to the favorite expression I found during my doctoral studies: "Velvet paradigmatic rut." How smooth and slick it is for us to slip down into our familiar, though not accurate, rut or samskara of seeing and thinking objects instead of relationships. It's only been over time that I've discovered how critical this specific point of discernment of relationships is to how I understand yoga. Allow me to describe why that rut serving as the avidyâ (ignorance) of objects leads us directly to asmitâ and the rest of the kleshas of suffering.

This big clod of objectification, or making things objects, generates the illusion of separateness. There is this, and there is that, both are separate and distinct. We come by this way of thinking for a variety of reasons including the European Enlightenment and the development of the modern scientific method. Both brought great utility and change to the world, but they also have the dark side of creating violence and harm by being disjunctive or separating while our ability to see relationships is lost or never well developed. As yoga professionals, this point about reductionism/parts is often presented when the concept of bodymind duality is introduced. Included in such presentations are the negative effects that the duality has on health and medicine. But it's been my observation, and possibly yours as well, that, beyond that, is about where the distinction ends. Pick up most any yoga book or DVD, or attend a workshop on yoga for any condition, and the objects are back. (Let's just pretend that we aren't included in that group for now.)

The condition is one object, the student with the condition is another object, the yoga prescription is a series of objects to apply to the other objects, and the advertised result (relief) is the final object. Link the objects together for relief of suffering and be sure to sign up for the follow-on courses to gain more objects. It is the figurative water we swim in and so very difficult to see real time as it's unfolding. And, when the recipe fails, we're off shopping for the next object to manipulate or use to "do to." That includes this book by the way. So, what are we to do to begin to change our lens of understanding from objects to relationships? Just like the old farmer, break up one clod after the other, over and over in clodhopper asana. Consider the following clod-busting activities.

Spotting Objects and Discovering Relationships

Discovering relationships and spotting objects is a skill. As with any skill, our performance improves with practice, feedback, and adaptation. Our relationship-seeing muscles are puny and underdeveloped from lack of practice. The remainder of this book is designed to gently, but regularly, begin to enhance our performance to realize the yoked/yoga of relationship reality in our experience and in the circumstances of those we serve. There isn't an endpoint or a final stopping point to this process of development. We're in this for the duration as far as I can see. In this chapter, we'll deconstruct some old clods and point to resources and activities that making the hopping a bit more effective.

(Did you know even the word clodhopper, which described the relationship between the farmer and the earth, was later modified to describe just the sturdy shoe and big foot as an object or clodhopper? This objectification is everywhere, I'm telling you.)

Yoga Lore and His-Story

We are fortunate to be living in an era of fresh investigation into the origins of yoga. Much of what was known of yoga in Western society was dependent on old British writings by male authors that lacked the context and historical archives modern scholars now have at their disposal. These modern authors also have a much broader view, drawing from historic artifacts, social and anthropological resources to, guess what? You got it, highlight relationships we weren't aware of, but influenced our earlier limited understandings and teachings about yoga. These inquiries haven't just been all sweetness and light, however. Many of our best stories about some romanticized Eden-like tale of this fully coherent, integrated, 5000-year-old tradition have been shattered. In the destruction of these tales has been the birth of a much richer, context-sensitive description of the weave of oral tradition, historical scholarship, socio and anthropological relationships, and our modern adoptions to these many and varied practices lumped under the object label of a "yoga" (Horton 2012; Mallinson and Singleton 2017; Schnäbele 2010; Singleton 2010).

Further clouding our limited understanding of yoga is the historical absence of women's voices, their contributions, and their more recent role in the understanding of yoga. How could we imagine ever understanding yoga as "relationships" without half of the human race? The more recent works of Gates (2006), Schnäbele (2010), and Horton (2012), are great resources for deepening our understanding of yoga to become more accurate and inclusive. Their work is every bit as scholarly and rigorous as the male-dominated descriptions of yoga history. Finally, yoga is no longer a his-story, as the deconstruction of the various fields illuminates for us. Instead, we begin to glimpse an expanding, ever-changing kaleidoscope of new relationships that inform our understanding of yoga.

Through this continuing spectrum of filters, what we think of as asana, breath control, yogic bodies, bandhas, mantra, withdrawal, meditation, and samadhi are all shift and shimmer in the light of investigation. If you have not read any of this work, I urge you to pick at least one of the above citations for further study. Each are extensively cited with references for deeper inquiry, while revealing different facets of the same "yoga" we thought we understood. At the start of this chapter I challenged you with some questions about the certainty of your understanding of yoga. These resources will surely turn over the soil of knowing and help create a fine new seed bed for new growth as we progress through this book. Just as in the days of the single plow share, poor soil preparation will lead to poor yields as new insights and concepts bounce off or lie buried beneath the hard pack of your knowing.

More Clods

For now, here's a partial list of concepts to break things up, and later you can read more deeply in the referenced works:

1. Your asana practice isn't hundreds of years old (probably barely a hundred years old at best).

2. Your lineage isn't "The" authentic lineage (they are many, sometimes related, and often of varied origins), so please stop marketing yourself as an authentic yoga master.

3. Your fourth chakra might not be blue (tremendous variation and conjecture around subtle yoga anatomy and how it might relate to Tantric yoga).

4. Was Patanjali an individual or a group of individuals (jury is still out)?

5. The focus on asana is a new thing (this one you probably knew) and is only mentioned four times in Patanjali's Yoga Sutras. Why is that?

6. Group classes isn't the way it's always been.

7. Corporate sponsorship is not just a new phenomenon in modern yoga. And the sponsors influenced those "pure" ancient practices.

8. Which liberation are you after? Yes, there are many described, so you should know which one to choose, right?

9. Duality or non-duality? But that's a duality, isn't it? Dang!

10. What's with all the realized [sic] lechers in modern yoga practice? Does that bother you like it does me?

11. How's the internet related to yoga? You hesitated…too slow. It is, but there aren't any books about it yet.

12. What will yoga look like in 20 years? You can't guess and neither can I. All we can presume is it will be very different and therefore is not a static entity.

13. If you are already whole and complete now, why do yoga? What's to be fixed? How do you keep it from breaking again if it wasn't right? Will you stay around to help the rest of us or are you out of here? This might sound a bit snarky, but liberation is the endgame if you read or study at many schools.

14. Which of the major yoga philosophies are right and how does that right one relate to Western philosophy? And do we just get rid of Western philosophy, then? Gulp.

15. Finally, how many yogis does it take to screw in a light bulb? Answer: zero. The light comes from within. Have I made my point? This last question might be a bad joke, but if you look back over the others with a bit of humility, can you sense the humor in each of those as well? We so want some certainty.

My working collection of relationships trying to define yoga is something like this: Yoga is evolving, not static. It is a process, not a conclusion, more verb than noun. More a personal relationship than an idea. More an experience than a dogma. Yoga invites us to experience the energy (the ability to do work) and action of relationships in an unending, unfolding process.

I share that collection because I realize that the list above may be a bit disturbing on some level. Probably even more disturbing later, when we describe the influence of modern inquiry through neuroscience, psychology, physiology, anatomy, and cosmology on our understanding of yoga. Rest assured that inquiry *will* further fine-comb the clods of what we know and can know, period, not just about yoga. We will save that for later chapters.

Before we move on, I find some comfort in Richard Rohr's (2013) perspective on relationships and Mystery, with a big "M." Fr. Rohr is a progressive, non-dual Franciscan priest true to the integral nature of St. Francis. Rohr claims that reality is radically relational, and all the power is in the relationships. He illustrates that by noting the power is not in the particles of atoms or the planets, but in the space in between the particles and planets. It sounds a lot like what we called the prana. He suggests that the only response before that invisible Mystery is immense humility, much like astrophysicists who are comfortable with darkness, emptiness, non-explainability (dark matter, black holes). He suggests the value of being OK in the Mystery is that it leaves us in many ways as a "stranger and pilgrim" on this earth, or, as we say, with a beginner's mind. Surrendering that certainty around what yoga is becomes a practice of great spiritual importance.

As long as we're uncomfortable, let's now consider the tricky topic of sorting out the differences between plain old garden-variety yoga [sic] and yoga therapy for additional clod busting. For that we need a new subheading.

What's the Deal with Yoga and Yoga Therapy?

We must address this difference because "yoga therapy" is in the title of the book. Why not just say "yoga as a creative response"? That's a good and fair question. The short answer: You technically could. But that doesn't leave us with much of a book. Plus, the difference in terminology is important within the rich context and relationships of modern life. Allow me to explain further.

I was fortunate to serve on the committee of the International Association of Yoga Therapy that drafted the first community-driven, official definition of yoga therapy back in 2005–2007 (Taylor 2007b). The committee was tasked to study, seek broad current and historical input from the international yoga community, and support dialog and consensus on a definition of yoga therapy. This task was part of a long process of development for the profession of yoga therapy. The first professional association conference known as SYTAR (Symposium of Yoga Therapy and Research) was held in 2007 in Los Angeles, CA. During the conference, numerous leaders presented and discussed their perspective of what constituted yoga therapy. The 600+ attendees listened and discussed as well, as we collected their input to add to our other research. It was only after all that effort that we sat down to use a qualitative, thematic process of constructing a functional definition. Such a definition is the foundation of any profession: What are you? There were also increasing inquiries from the press, the public, and researchers seeking to understand what this yoga therapy stuff is anyway. There was also the increasing likelihood of legal requests for definition as more people were putting themselves out as yoga therapists. We will get to the definition shortly, but some more context is important.

The yoga clod of modern yoga is often built squarely on Patanjali Sutra 1.2:

> *Yogash citta vrtti nirodha*: Yoga is the cessation/stabilization of the modifications, or fluctuations, of the mind.

Of the nearly 5000 yoga schools registered with the Yoga Alliance in the USA, if there is any one consensus definition, it would be some version of that sutra or the more colloquial "yoga = union or yoking." I have reviewed depositions on yoga injury cases as an expert witness, and this is the best that comes forward in training manuals and testimony. Needless to say, it means almost nothing legally and sure doesn't explain the modern postural yoga business with the emphasis on asana. But even this clod of a definition as a sutra succumbs to its own vrittis with scrutiny to the point that the packed dirt becomes fine sand of uncertainty slipping through our fingers. Amazon's around 3000 returns for "yoga sutra" is a good first clue.

Granted they aren't all sutra commentaries, something is going on with hundreds of books published to illuminate the meaning of the sutras. We won't belabor the point about a solid definition, but if you haven't gone deeply into that single sutra, I'd recommend Crisfield's blog post (2017) as a good starting point for deconstructing your clod. I checked with several scholars, and as expected, the consensus was "pretty accurate, but…" each with a different "but"!

Crisfield begins by describing how each of the three words besides yogash have broad and varied definitions that don't easily translate from Sanskrit and of course also have different historical contexts from today. Her thick description of each and how the qualities interact in multiple paradoxes leaves the reader with something far different than "Yoga stills the mind." Critical to what we'll be talking about later in this chapter is the nature of the yoga concepts of manas and buddhi, and how the latter gives rise naturally and appropriately to a sense of separate self, which then generates asmitâ. But that's OK, as they are one small part of the play and relationship within citta of self and Self, both of which are part of the movement of vrittis that aren't to be frozen or fixed, but known from the stillness of the seer, which sets up another paradox of movement and stillness with no separation between us and the world. Phew! So, the sutra describes the integral and paradoxical relationships between the words describing complex relationships versus a mechanistic (our culture's dominant model) of someone (object) holds something (a different object) still which makes yoga (another object). Yikes.

The takeaway of all of this is to suggest that I, and, I'm betting, you, can't with words only define yoga conclusively. Hence the realization (to make real) only comes about from practice and lived experience, not conceptually. Therefore, we also can't teach "yoga" with words because what that experience of yoga in the student is will have to be different for each of them based on their unique lived experience and their narrative around such experiences. Yoga is not stuff we give (a commodity) to another. We merely create an environment for the other to experience something and integrate that experience into their life. Quite a contrast from detailed asana instruction and demonstration with the successful end product being the performance of a movement that allows one to check one more off on their asana life list. That which I just described is instruction, an object-oriented activity of doing to get something, not the relational quality of yoga of the second sutra described above. Instruction is very different from education (*educare*: to draw out from within) where the insight to relationships emerges. Much more later, just keep clear on the difference between instruction and education. That's my instruction.

Did I forget to also mention the many present-day misconceptions around what is marketed as yoga as further confusing our understanding of what is yoga? Ask the average person on the street (and most personal injury attorneys) and they say something about the twisty-bendy acrobatics classes as being yoga. If they're particularly aware, they might confess to not quite understanding how the goats, beer, funky music, or paddleboards fit into yoga! I have extended this discussion around the definition of yoga to hopefully soften up your certainty, but also to illustrate the confused state of the term yoga when the International Association of Yoga Therapists (IAYT) decided to formalize the term yoga therapy. Formalizing the term established the profession of yoga therapy as being distinct from yoga. So, let's now explore what we came up with and why it's important for serving those in pain. (Hint: It might also ease some of our suffering too.)

What Means Yoga Therapy?

I admit that subtitle is bad English. I use the expression because of my personal history with vocabulary and my affection for words. My dad loved to tell the story of how after parent–teacher conferences in my second grade, they returned home and told me how the teacher had said what a tremendous vocabulary I had for a second grader. To which I replied, "What means, 'vocabulary'?" Let's take that same innocent, honest inquiry into what means yoga therapy.

The foundational definition was carefully wordsmithed by our committee. A much more extensive definition is now also available on the website (www.iayt.org) but this definition was the original and still serves as a succinct means of communicating within our culture to consumers, researchers, media, legal entities, and yoga professionals:

> Yoga therapy is the process of empowering individuals to progress toward improved health and wellbeing through the application of the teachings and practices of Yoga. (Taylor 2007b, p.3)

Allow me to share some of the meticulous word selection that I believe helps to differentiate our very messy modern definition of yoga from yoga therapy. *Process* reinforces that yoga therapy is not an event, do this and that is then fixed. Process reflects an ongoing set of relational changes forged by both philosophical conceptual change *and* the changes from practice brought about by the many yoga technologies that are available. The test for whether it is yoga therapy is dependent on the level of empowerment experienced by the student. If the process is not *empowering*, but leaves the person dependent on teacher, technique, or some other power holder, it isn't yoga therapy. *Toward* is the intention and it is directional, but not about treating diseases or curing conditions. That's the role of other professions. Yoga therapy gives the person power as they discover/realize their innate true being within the therapeutic process versus something being done to or for them. This realization is *health*, and that realization is what provides a sense of *wellbeing* whether they are a young child or terminally ill in active transition.

The *application* of both *teachings and practices* holds the tension not just of doing a technique for relief, but having the context of self-understanding transformed beyond the individual's usual conditioned state. That alteration is what dispels misperceptions/vrittis that lead to suffering. Wild thing asana executed without any self-concept modification isn't yoga therapy, and neither is rote memorization of the sutras without enactment of the principles into one's daily behaviors. There must be both. The application of *teachings*/philosophy does not mean adherence to some dogmatic ideology, but the study and application of the perennial principles of the yamas, niyamas, and additional applicable yogic texts in such a way that they empower the individual within their unique life circumstance. This *application* exposes the possibility for new relationships, or reveals old relationships that aren't *healthy* and detract from *wellbeing*. This individual is now able to observe and evaluate those relationships in an ongoing *process* (life?) of constant experience, reflection, and new action. It is this cycle that fosters creative responses, but we are getting ahead of ourselves talking about creativity.

Therefore, yoga therapy shouldn't be about going to consume a product/treatment/class as a remedy to fix something. That's the other health models. Might a yoga therapy session or class generate some symptom improvement? Quite possibly, but that isn't the purpose or intent. The yoga therapy creates the environment and space for discovery and exploration of both true self nature and those misperceptions that are causing or will cause suffering. Therapists will differ in their ability to create such environments, but the therapist isn't the healing agent and dependence on a guru-type intervention leaves the individual disempowered.

Can you sense how this might not be the actual way yoga therapy is branded or marketed in your experience? Is that a problem? Am I off base about your skills or those of your teacher? It's OK to be a bit uncomfortable right now. Bear with me. While this isn't a book of techniques to apply for some predicted outcome or fix, I hope you are also glimpsing that maybe, just maybe, there's something deeper that is worth exploring. I believe there is. Now that we don't know what yoga is, but do know what yoga therapy is (that's a joke), some review and refreshed exploration of ethics will give us a new foundation to rebuild our understanding of yoga (and of course yoga therapy).

I Exercise My Ethics Plenty, Thanks

I have never heard yoga defined in a discussion as a "psychospiritual technology" in 20 years of study and yoga related organizational leadership. Yet, that is arguably how one of the greatest Western yoga scholars to have lived, Georg Feuerstein, defined yoga (Feuerstein 1998). Odd, there's no mention of where my knee should be in relation to my big toe in that definition? Rather, this definition suggests the importance of psychological and spiritual inquiry as the bedrock of yoga. That then brings us to ask, how do ethics, a key component of both inquires, relate to pain and suffering? I want to explore that question a good deal here, as ethics have not been the focus of modern yoga and yoga therapy teaching, but ought to be front and center of a new, emerging understanding of both. Don't worry though, this isn't a lecture on being good and the rules to keep you good. Fortunately, colleagues have recently published an important perspective article on the topic that is very exciting and practical (Sullivan *et al.* 2017). The article was just like finding that critical jigsaw puzzle piece that allows you to fill in an entire section of blue sky.

Sullivan *et al.* (2017) presented a framework of understanding that bridges classic ethical and philosophical yoga to modern research and healthcare. The article goes far beyond "Being good is good for you." I strongly encourage you to find the article and read it in its entirety. A brief summation is woven into our discovery process, but it by no means conveys the richness of their work. Later in Chapter 3 on wisdom we will expand on the importance of including these central existential issues in our teaching.

In Chapter 4 on pain we will get into details of how the Upanishads, the Bhagavad Gita, the Samkhya Karika, the Yoga Sutras, and the Hatha Yoga Pradipika provide guidance and practices to transform students' perspectives and ultimately alleviate suffering. These are the classic *teachings* mentioned in the yoga therapy definition. Our ability to offer yoga therapy with a culturally familiar explanation of the teachings and practices is going to be essential in our effectiveness in the world. Such an explanation will allow you to improve your therapeutic reasoning skills, communicate with other healthcare providers, and gain acceptance from potential clients, providers, organizations, and researchers (Sullivan *et al.* 2017). Don't let research be an obstacle. Research (re-search: to look again) is just our modern and dominant form of inquiry into reality. As such it has its own drawbacks and limitations, but there are also some newer, more robust and exciting methods that are gaining strength because of their ability to address complex phenomena such as pain and suffering. The authors share four methods: phenomenology, eudaimonia, virtue ethics, and first-person ethical inquiry. Becoming familiar with them is worth the effort. Here we go.

When you listen to your student's responses to situations during an intake, you are practicing a form of *phenomenology*. When you pay attention and value their personal report (first-person) of their thoughts, emotions, embodied actions, and social interactions that process generates a research for both of you into understanding the meaning around their suffering. The searching often leads to insights as to how their body, mind, and environment (BME) are related. There's relationships again. Layered with those relationships of course is awareness as our true nature (Purusha) with the BME (Prakriti) that is both the cause of suffering and the means of easing and preventing suffering. Paradoxes too. This intake inquiry and feedback during subsequent teachings and practices reveals ever more accurate perceptions of the connections of relationship between the BME and awareness, leading to creative new possible actions to alleviate suffering. We will return to creative responses in the creativity chapter, but, for now, you are a budding phenomenologist. Congratulations. Provided you both are discovering *their* understanding, not you directing what they should understand, of course.

The key point to keep in mind is, as this fabric of relationships becomes clearer through teachings and practices, clarity is the result of the student's lived, embodied experience, not some passive thinking process. Their intertwined relationships are brought into focus through awareness and that becomes the foundation from which they can move *toward wellbeing*. They also discover their habitual patterns of movement, intentions, and ways of engaging their environment (samskaras). These discoveries reorient their identity away from the misperceptions (vrittis) of the BME, which then primes them to change their meaning and purpose accordingly. In other words, the person is *empowered* to change their relationship to the nature of suffering that is occurring in their experience because of their own inquiry versus someone else's prescription of what their next actions should be. This process of active engagement yields shared decision making with their care team and a new, or enhanced, experience of agency around their suffering. This empowerment of understanding their habits and creating new responses is called discriminative wisdom and we will explore it in more detail in Chapter 3 on wisdom. For now, appreciate how yoga therapy is a very practical application that can *empower* individuals to have new choices in their own discovery *process*.

It is important for us to move away from treating or battling the diagnoses, and instead have our and our students' focus on the lived experience and how that lived experience restructures identity and orientation of the BME. People suffering report many challenges in the BME to include: the body as alien; powerless; isolated; rejecting or distancing from the affected body part; an unraveling of identity; disorientation, uncertainty, loss of familiarity with their body; an inability to engage with the world as they had before; an altered sense of identity; an increased attention to bodily function; that their body is no longer experienced in the background or as transparent when engaging life; lacking a harmony within the BME; and the world sometimes feels diminished (Sullivan *et al.* 2017). We will get to how yoga therapy is a methodology for addressing those reports later in the book, but first, what is *wellbeing* and how is it related to ethics?

By our operating definition, yoga therapy is a movement toward *health* and *wellbeing*. As yoga therapists, we're to create environments that allow the student to experience qualities such as calm, joy, peace, or contentment, irrespective of the source of the suffering. The social media groups are full of yoga professionals seeking to address the diagnosis of a person, indicating they've missed this important point that distinguishes yoga therapy from the other practices. Certainly, when we succeed in creating experiences where those qualities are experienced the person can also experience symptom relief from their diagnosis as well. But that isn't our focus. Do you know the fancy modern word for what our focus as yoga therapists should be?

It is *eudaimonia*. This Greek word that Aristotle used describes a flourishing and enduring form of happiness. Not a transient, pleasurable experience, but a deeper, lasting joy or bliss, to use our yoga language. Don't worry about remembering the word, but know that there is modern research that relates to it as an outcome and explores what behaviors leads to the experience. Search "bliss" or "ananda" and you won't find anything in research literature. Eudaimonia is the modern word to search. There currently is a long list of positive health benefits we all know from yoga practice that also includes decreased social isolation and increased presence of meaning in one's life. In Chapter 4 on pain we explore this more deeply for its importance. My purpose in including it now is that it is the often overlooked practices of the yamas and niyamas that provide a method for altering identity, generating meaning and purpose, as well experiencing eudaimonia. There's the bridge!

Regarding the third research method, *virtue ethics*, Sullivan *et al.* (2017) write:

> The practice of ethical investigation reflects an exploration of how one holds a system of values or beliefs about right or wrong and good or bad, informing one's decisions and actions towards a well-intentioned life. One's ethical framework forms the context for inquiry into life's experiences, such as illness, and serves as the foundation from which action and meaning are created. (epub ahead of print)

The exploration of this foundation is essential prior to generating what in yoga we describe as "right action" and one's dharma or right path in life. When grounded in an ethical practice, the aspiration is to benefit both the student and society as directed by not only Aristotle (Garchar 2012), but Sri Aurobindo in his integral yoga philosophy (Aurobindo 1993). Remember this inclusion of "society" when we move into the next chapter.

What is important for now is that the modern term for this practice is the last method the authors described. The term is *first-person ethics* and represents a phenomenological approach of inquiry or research. See how this all ties together? As I promised, this form of ethics isn't a study of outer moral judgment or rules to follow, but a "subjective and intentional experience of ethics that helps to align one's thoughts, feelings, and actions" (Sullivan *et al.* 2017). The intention is *toward* eudaimonia or a well-lived life and it is acted out through the BME as actions. It is through this approach an understanding of the transformative nature of the suffering can be illuminated to include any changes in identity. This active form of engagement is critical when dealing with a persistent pain or health challenge as the person's BME will change and require an empowered individual to refine their understanding through actions across a lifetime rather than a one-time fix. Such an active engagement in their own care encourages the student to redefine the many relationships to the challenge, and these reevaluations will be key in living with the complexities of chronic pain as we'll see later. (Hint: the intention of moving toward eudaimonia will cast a harsh light on the ridiculousness of the present day cultural drive for unsustainable consumption.)

With gratitude to the authors (Sullivan *et al.* 2017) for weaving this together, we are now in a position to move on to the next chapter. Presumably that solid ground of knowing what yoga is has been tilled and prepared for the fascinating implications of our new, not-so-certain fluid definition of yoga and the related profession of yoga therapy. If we try to create from the same place we have always been, odds are that not much new or practical is going to come forward. The deeper we dig, the more we turn over around our assumptions and beliefs, the more we will be primed to be the change agents our profession asks of us.

Give yourself the gift of reflection on this chapter and write down your answers to these questions before continuing. (Jot them down versus just thinking them.) What did this chapter shift in your working definition of yoga? What do you want to explore more of from our discoveries? Anything resurrected that you used to know but had set aside? (Jot them down.) How are you doing with this book not being a "do this for that" set of directions? What concerns you about that? (Make some notes.) Maybe you are just relieved and excited?

Now let's head into the next chapter to dive deep into many more "So whats?"

We are after all, you and I, are on an aspirational journey toward eudaimonia as well.

> We discover an older unity. My dear brothers and sisters, we are already one. But we imagine that we are not. So what we have to recover is our original unity. What we have to be is what we are. (Thomas Merton, cited in Fox 2016, p.62)

2

. . .

Implications from the
New Yoga Therapy

MINNESOTA ADVENTURE

My first yoga teacher, Jeff Wright, taught from an Iyengar style. Very precise and detailed in explanation and execution. His primary modality was asana practice with some occasional pranayama instruction. Reflecting on the experience, I don't recall him ever instructing us in the yamas and niyamas. At least not directly. I now appreciate that he taught them by his behavior and lifestyle. Honest, humble, content, joyful, and non-grasping. There was something attractive about his simple kindness that spoke volumes more than any lecture ever could. Of course, early on I just consumed every bit of technical asana expertise I could garner from him and then, as I began to study, even resented his teaching style as too rigid or inflexible for me, the new yoga guy all about connection and love for all (I thought). Ah, the same headstrong patterns that threw my spine in a knot weren't so easy to unravel despite the relief of the back pain. In retrospect, I can now appreciate how many more layers had yet to fall away back then. Today I can glimpse many more that will need to die as my practice continues.

. . .

Up in the cabin I just wanted pain relief. Today, I just want pain relief. Not a relief of a bodily type pain at present. The pain today is that output from my BME that warns me of the challenges ahead in our world. Not some paranoid, Doomsday perspective, but the result of the double-edged sword of extended practice and wisdom. This integral perspective we are examining doesn't solve a "thing," rather it uses each lesson to prep for the next. My yoga practice didn't end when my back stabilized, it just had me prepared for the next tougher lesson. Sorry. Seems to be the deal. So, let's have some fun discovering what's next in our yoga therapy now that we've destroyed our old understandings. It's a *process*, in a direction. We aspire to ease present suffering and prevent future suffering.

Last chapter we broke up some of the hard-packed soil of certainty about how we define yoga. We also introduced a working definition of yoga therapy as a contrast to standard yoga instruction. All of which is fine, but if it didn't suggest new behavior changes for us as yoga professionals, what would be the point? Describing new possible behaviors is the reason for this chapter: Make it useful, Taylor. In order for the ever-changing, evolving yoga and yoga therapy to thrive in our newly tilled soil of uncertainty and change, there ought to be some practical implications to harvest. Hop on our epistemological combine and let's see what is ready for harvest.

Our First-Person Ethics Review

We begin now with our fresh perspective about the importance of the phenomenological process of a first-person ethics review in yoga therapy. Our self-identity should literally change through such an inquiry as to whether our behavior matches our intention to live by the yamas and niyamas. Do we take right actions to fulfill those intentions? This review is our work first, prior to resuming working with students. I want to begin our harvest of implications by choosing one low-hanging fruit that is woven into the heart of both the yamas and our yoga therapy definition. That fruit is the first yama of ahimsâ (non-harming) and how it relates to *the process of empowering individuals*. If we mess up this one, game over for our yoga therapy relieving suffering for the other, or ourselves. As an expert witness for yoga injuries, I'm not talking about stupid (the only word that describes the behavior in most cases that have retained me) or gross negligent behavior that causes harm. The harm I'm referencing is nearly invisible and I'm as guilty as the next yoga therapist of having violated this yama.

What I've done and see going on in the name of yoga therapy is an unconscious slipping into our mechanistic society's worldview of what I call "doing to": offering linear recipes of yoga practice solutions. This occurs when we: (1) Don't take the time to allow the student to find the solution; (2) Don't give the process time to unfold and either literally or metaphorically push our agenda; (3) Tell the student how to think about, interpret, or integrate an insight to "fix" their suffering rather than creating the environment for them to find their way to their unique identity; (4) Assume to know who they are and what they want; and (5) a hundred or more other variations on those themes. I've written extensively on this topic (Taylor 2004, 2006, 2007a) because when we take the power away from the student we not only harm them, but we take the heart out of what the profession of yoga therapy can become, and we reinforce our own samskara of thinking we are the cause of healing. That samskara sets us up for future suffering as we become more attached to that self-image. A nasty trifecta of unintended harming.

Pause a moment and note your thoughts, emotions, and bodily response as you consider what I just wrote. Is there room for you to improve? Why would you want to change your behavior? Could any suffering you are experiencing around your current practice be tied to this principle? Note this shortcoming isn't just about you and your students. First and foremost, is this how you care for yourself in your personal practice? Can you hold any new insight in the soft light of an exciting discovery rather than the harsh light of interrogation? Such a realization (again, to make real) is a gift, not a moral condemnation. That's the power of our yogic first-person ethics review. A discovery of that type is the seed of new possibility we can plant for the relief of future suffering. But planting is only the next step. You may also feel the discomfort of the related implications. How do I not direct? Will the student find their way? What if the student doesn't come back? You know the litany. Let's just let that discomfort be for now. If we can begin to better support ourselves and our students with less harming, that is fantastic. As for the answers to these other concerns, well, that's why I need to keep typing.

Certainty Traps Are Everywhere

Don't be throwing off your clodhoppers just because we got that last chapter behind us. Creating clods of certainty is what we do. Going forward in this book please insert "maybe" at the end of every declarative sentence (except this one). We had to break up all those old clods of certainty to be primed for creating a better future. The last thing we want to do is start making more. There will be many exercises on how to recognize those clods in the practice chapter, but I want to warn you about the rest of this book. The current best trap is the use of "neuro": neurophysiology, neuroimaging, neuroscience, neuroplastics, neuroliberation… Well, I made up that last one, but it just might sell.

We will be discussing many concepts founded on just those words. Please take it all with a big grain of salt. It is another certainty trap. Check out the titles of yoga workshops, products, and keynote speeches. Neuro is everywhere. Am I saying there isn't utility or important insights to be gained from neuro-stuff? Not at all. But they're all subject to error in interpretation, reproducibility, and most of all, limited representation of complexity. It is beyond the scope of our discussion to fully describe all the limitations, so either take my word for it or search the topic on your own. For our purposes, just consider any claim with neuro is just as vulnerable to vrittis as any other claim. Let me illustrate my warning by sharing one fascinating little study addressing a yogic hard-packed idea.

You've probably heard or read that a yogic practice has been shown to increase the amount of time and ease with which you can generate alpha range waves in your brain. Scientists put sensors on a subject's skull, use an electroencephalogram to measure and document activity, comparing various groups. From those studies, we all "know" alpha wave = good: Do yoga: Get more alpha waves. Well, while this was not a peer-reviewed study, it had a large N (number of subjects) and they reported something interesting (Parameshwaran and Thiagarajan 2017). They found indications of relationship between alpha wave generation and an absence of ability to generate alpha waves in those subjects without post-primary education and access to modern technology. (Read:

environment:mind relationship.) To make matters even more slippery, those that did generate alpha waves did so with wide variation of over a thousandfold with no centralized mean. (There isn't "an" alpha wave to obtain, and what we called alpha waves varies tremendously.) And alpha waves are old by study standards with simple technology versus complex modern imaging. Yet, this study suggests no definitive outcomes of certainty and possibly that the context of a person's environment affects the ability to even generate such a pattern of electrical activity in the brain. The lesson: The "E" in BME is a powerful component of our lived experiences and doesn't reside in our brains/neuro.

My point here being, ignore the pretty colored images and always conclude reviewing a study with "maybe." That whole right-brain/left-brain that still gets sold has been tossed in the trash bin labeled "Not even kinda that simple folks." If you are teaching some "neuro" concept without qualifying yourself regularly as "not certain," you're creating clods that will need to be broken up later. Stop it please. Now, let me teach you some neuro.

Nervous System Fertilizer

Every sentence of this section, as with all the other sentences in this book, should end with "maybe." Please also note the euphemism in this section's title, remembering the most common farming source of fertilizer. There, now we are in the proper frame of mind.

The powerful lens of inquiry made possible by the scientific method are fascinating. The last 100+ years of looking deeply at the orders of parts, from the smallest bits to the far reaches of the cosmos, have revealed the same thing. That revelation is that there is an apparently unending horizon in all directions. The brightest minds on the planet agree that, not only are we limited as humans in our comprehension of reality, there is substantial argument for the possibility of multiple other realities. Oh, no, he's going to talk about quantum physics! Not to worry. I won't, because I don't understand it. I'm just making a point that, if the really smart people are having those types of discussions, the rest of us can be OK with just not being certain in our small, "solid" classical physics lives. There's enough here to mess with our minds, we don't need to pretend to understand the implications of quantum science because the scientists admit even they don't understand it. The good news is there's plenty of very cool stuff available on our level to evoke awe and for us to marvel at in wonder.

What I want to highlight in this section of implications is the concept of neuroplasticity. No, you can't change your nervous system to heal every disease or trauma that is creating suffering. Sorry. What is fascinating to me is that 37 years ago when I was learning neuroanatomy and neurophysiology the very concept was heresy. The nervous system is plastic (changeable)? There's some fertilizer. We were taught that in adulthood, the nervous system was what it was going to be and if you wrecked any of it through disease, injury, or poor lifestyle choices, there was no way to repair or change the new result. The only direction was downward to something less functional.

Fast forward to today, and the word is everywhere. Amazon lists over 500 books with the word in the title. That's a bunch of fertilizer. Seriously, there is some very good science that has demonstrated the nervous system can change in both function (how it works) and in structure (actual form). This is radical, changing the very foundations of our very limited understanding. Unfortunately, those finding are also spawning some pretty crazy claims from both qualified and unqualified salespeople. The lines are now blurred between scientists who write good books, scientists who write books so they will sell, and science journalists who cover the gamut, good to bad. In Chapter 4 on pain we will cover what I find practical about neuroplasticity for us as yoga professionals.

The implication I want to share here is how neuroplasticity breaks up so much of what we thought we knew about our nervous systems, which means we need to surrender our certainty about what is possible for healing and easing suffering. Not knowing what is possible into the future is only one outcome of the annihilation of certainty. Because the nervous system is adaptable across the lifespan, we also don't fully understand how environment and social relationships drive neurological function to create suffering and pain either. And more "bad" news for certainty seekers: It appears the nervous system, immune system, skeletal system, digestive system and the rest of them…well, they're all tied together and have powerful and direct influences on one another. Oh, one more thing. Apparently experience and environmental factors can generate heritable genetic functional changes and be passed through the functional expressions of genes. Isn't that amazing? Certainty crumbles in every direction we look and this "everything is relationships" stuff appears real in emerging science. It might just be accurate (maybe).

Before we move on, should all this uncertainty drive our plastic nervous systems to collapse? No, I believe it frees us from the rigidity related to a false certainty. This new-found flexibility and adaptability offers a stronger resilience for us to engage the uncertain future and will facilitate our creativity in solving present suffering and preventing future suffering. The next section introduces some ways our modern science reinvigorates our understanding of classical yoga principles. The section will also be a threshold for us to build a taxonomy (naming things and processes) and lexicon (the language to communicate effectively) for both our clients and our broader community of referral sources, administrators, philanthropists, and other influencers. Here we go.

(Did he really get through that section without mentioning mirror neurons? Almost.)

Is All That Is Old New Again?

Some of the new growth in yoga is the emergence of "old" yoga technologies. We already highlighted the relevance of the yamas and niyamas as one such sprout. In this section we will consider several more, as new options increase the likelihood for creative new expressions of our evolving yoga. I will also introduce two new terminologies that represent old yoga concepts just packaged in modern language. Our ability to identify these growths as part of our harvest and not weeds or distractions are important discernments. If we have too much tied up in a hard-packed definition of yoga, these sprouts will either be trampled or discarded as weeds. I'm inviting you to remain open and enjoy the exploration. The "risk" of including something that isn't yoga is significantly offset by the benefit of identify new varietals.

Kleshas: As Sullivan *et al.* (2017) did for the yamas and niyamas, it seems the kleshas might be next, as research findings into pain and suffering keep circling back to these five sources of suffering. The brilliance of the overarching first kleshas of avidyâ (ignorance) of not recognizing the interconnection of all of reality equates to much of what we will discuss in Chapter 3 on wisdom ahead. The other kleshas will be described later in this chapter. The simplicity of their composition and practical ability to identify sources of suffering are important to share with our students and to study their application in our lives as well. More to come, but you heard it here first when, ten years from now, everyone is using them.

Bandhas: How often do you use the bandhas in your teaching? Do you believe your students receive much practical application for them in their daily lives? Funny story, but a practical aid for we teachers. I could never quite remember how to spell bandhas and was going to teach a workshop that included them. When I Googled the term the second finding was a picture of Led Zeppelin standing in front of their jet in the 1970s. Being my favorite band, that got my attention. Here the person writing that post had made a typo, "The bandhas a jet of their own." I haven't forgotten how to spell bandhas since, and now neither will you.

There's even more utility to bandhas though. I appreciate that classically bandhas are described as powerful but subtle energetic realities that with study and practice lead to enhanced wellbeing and progression toward liberation. But did you know the location of those bandhas "coincidentally" lie right where modern movement researchers describe three related areas that need to be integrated to generate what they describe as "state of the art postural control"? Further, loss of integration of these three areas from disease, trauma, or lack of awareness not only creates faulty movement, but ties into how one breathes, the state of the autonomic nervous system, and the life narrative the person then authors as a result. I replicated the 15-minute "talk" I gave every new student the past 13 years of my practice because it was so profoundly useful in them beginning to understand the yoga of their complaints. (You can watch it at www.3diaphragms.com.) Something old is new again, and fun to teach.

Vayus: You do vayu, do you? The sages' descriptions of these five "energetic" descriptors of prana can be a bit intimidating given their Sanskrit names and the fact that most new students can perceive at most one, maybe a second one. And "So what?" they might ask. Turns out there's a big reason. When we attend to the perception of the vayus, we are activating old, deep structures of our thalamus (I like to call it Thelma-mess, students can remember it better). These representational maps were discovered by Dr. A. D. "Bud" Craig (2015), a functional neuroanatomist. This area of the brain could be where emotions arise as well as our sense of time and eudaimonia. As we will describe later, both compassion and creativity depend on affective regulation and awareness. Maybe (see I'm using maybe) regular attention to our affect (to include sensing the vayus) also modifies our ability to accurately feel our emerging state and have choices about taking new possible actions? His discoveries are quite recent, so no studies have been conducted on yoga applications and this is just conjecture on my part, based on what else we've observed in other areas. Either way, looking inward to study what we find is making looking at vayus not so esoteric and having very practical implications. I can just feel it.

Mudras: Related to vayus, the inward attention to changes in perception might stop some of the silly magical qualities being sold as mudras for ingrown toenails. The relationships between mudras, generally addressing hand positons, but including other bodily seals, and what we pay attention to, is valuable. Craig's (2015) subtitle is "An Interoceptive Moment with Your Neurobiological Self." I know I cautioned you about "neuro" but my guess is that we will find some interesting correlations/relationships between mudras and our interoceptive skills and how that affects our feelings (pun intended). Nora Bateson (2017) does an amazing job of deconstructing what we think a hand is as an object versus as a relational understanding of that part of the body as an interface between our interior and exterior experiences. (Hint: they aren't just mechanical claws for grasping and picking.) I recommend exploring mudras yourself if they aren't a regular part of your practice, not looking to manifest a new BMW, but discovering in more detailed nuances your interior experience. I have a feeling you will enjoy it.

Indryas: Are you familiar with this yogic concept of our senses, the five in and five outward senses? They were articulated out of the Kashmiri Shaivism period (Feuerstein 1998). Basically it was a model of the interaction between the interior and exterior sensations out of which our interaction with the rest of the world arises. Guess what? We have an exciting new [sic] model from the neuroscientists that illustrates the relationships involved in our body–self neuromatrix (see, put neuro and matrix together and it sounds real). They've discovered that there are things they call inputs (jnanendryas?) and outputs (karmendriyas?) that continually change across the flow of time, all of which construct a human being's identity/sense of self. Search both body–self neuromatrix and indriyas and marvel at the old becoming new again, with words and language our culture can understand. If indriyas didn't make sense before, they should now. Empowered with the language of our culture you can communicate with any group in a way they can consider and then experience with your directed practice of the principles. First try it on yourself. Just fascinating.

Chant and mantra: What percentage of your students regularly use chant or mantra for relief of their suffering? I suspect not many…yet. There's so much exciting science being explored in this area of human sound production, and yet beyond occasional kirtan experiences, and maybe a single word mantra, these technologies are grossly underutilized in modern yoga practice. Granted there needs to be a cultural sensitivity to the person's belief structures and making chants and mantras accessible from a language acquisition perspective. I also know the yoga purists will assert that Sanskrit in its magnificent construction brings what sound like magical powers. I hear you. I'd also like to have you read Craig's work and then resume your practice. There's a goldmine there. Note not only the way the practices modify and increase the maps of your "body–self neuromatrix," but also integrate the three diaphragms in both perception and performance affecting postural stability and oral/glottal/diaphragmatic recruitment. See how the fancy modern language feels compared to the allegorical description of affecting the flow of the nadis, opening chakras, engaging jalandhara, and releasing the kundalini? Both are accurate, just the size of the audience shifts dramatically. Especially if you further modify it to something like "Varying the sounds you produce through your vocal chords, the movement of your diaphragm, and then how those sounds create a powerful relaxation response while you upgrade your google-map resolution for movement planning is exciting!" Have fun dressing up the old in new clothing.

BPS(S) and panca maya koshas: I am presuming most of you are familiar with the panca maya kosha model, long described from the Upanishads, of the five interwoven sheaths of human experience: anna, prâna, mano, vijnâna, and ananda. Now try selling that to a physician, administrator, or conservative student. See the problem? Once again, conventional medicine is pumped up because they are beginning to approach patients in a bio-psycho-social (BPS) framework. They're still pretty squeamish about the parenthetical second "S," spirit. Who knew all these parts of human experience were interrelated? Uhm, maybe the Taittiriya-Upanishad from around the sixth century bce (Feuerstein 1998)? As the hubris of the scientific model wanes, the second "S" will get added. We already have reliable and validated measurement scales for spirituality, but it still seems a bit too subjective for many 'serious' scientists or providers. And when it happens, there will be much congratulatory back-slapping around their important new finding that spirit matters.

One of the koshas of course deserves a moment in the spotlight: vijnâna. While mano simply coordinates sensory input, vijnâna is understanding, a higher cognitive function according to Feuerstein (1998). This quality of consciousness in the vijnâna sheath would later be spotlighted in Vasabandhu's Vijnânavâda and for Vedanta philosophers as the big "C," universal Consciousness or ultimate reality (Feuerstein 1998, p.230). The perennial quest for this consciousness of various descriptions leads to this kosha as frequently described as the "wisdom" body. There will be much more to say about wisdom in the next chapter.

Mindsphere: You probably haven't heard of this one yet, unless you read Siegel (2017). Mindsphere may never catch on, but I include it as an example of unearthing an old yogic concept and putting new words to describe the concept in our modern context. I use it a few more times in the book as it reinforces many of the principles I'm sharing here. What is it? We are comfortable with atmosphere, both literal and metaphorically. Biosphere makes sense too, correct? Where life is found in, on and around the earth. What do you call the atmosphere of energy and information flow that surrounds us and shapes our reality? Siegel calls it mindsphere (2017). When you read his definition of mind below in the *Word Choice* section it will make even more sense. For now, just consider how this relates to the interpersonal, transcendent nature of the various yogic descriptions of the many facets of mind (mana, buddhi, citta, etc.) and Aurobindo's supermind of integral yoga philosophy. The words we choose matter so much. Can we bring our profession forward by teaching from the present mindsphere that is familiar and safe to those who are already overwhelmed by pain and suffering, without asking them to dive into foreign spheres? I think so and I hope you are having fun doing so right now.

What other old to new yoga concepts or teachings can you find? They're everywhere. That's one of the things that is so remarkable about yoga: Anything new has probably been described somewhere in yoga. Our task as yoga professionals is to have the jnana rigor to seek and bridge the new back through the old, and then have it make sense and become practical to ourselves and those we serve. Another tool for us is to develop our ability to say it so the most people can make good use of it.

Say It for the Most

One observation I have about yoga professionals in general is that we haven't been very good at communicating what we do in a way most people can even understand, let alone relate to. The implication then from our new and evolving understanding of yoga and yoga therapy is that to be effective we need to dramatically improve our communication ability. We have harvested the low-hanging fruit of those who will try anything. We've also accessed the part of the next segment of the market that will try something new based on a warm referral of someone they have a great deal of confidence in that suggests they try yoga. That covers at most about 25–30 percent of the market. How are we going to reach the rest? I think we need to: (1) Develop multiple ways of explaining the benefits of what we do; (2) Those explanations need to match the vocabulary and worldview of the intended audience; (3) Read across multiple disciplines (not just the yoga world) to discover already overlapping areas of interest and practice in other disciplines and then invite collaboration; and (4) Bring our message to the venues and platforms that offer the best leverage for earning acceptance and us being identified as thought leaders (media, conferences, workshops, local support groups, etc.).

I understand that's a tall order. If I had a penny for every word I edit for simplicity in just this book I could take a great vacation. I'm right there with you needing to improve. In this section I want to share some examples of people who are communicating that way and demonstrate some ways we can all do the four steps above. With those examples, I hope you will follow suit and begin finding examples or creating your own. There'll be many exercises around this principle in the practice chapter. Enjoy this selection of ways to bridge to our current culture. This won't be exhaustive, but I think inspirational, and fuel for you to contribute to the future clarity of communications from yoga professionals.

Word Choice

Do you keep a collection of useful words to share what you teach? The words we choose can either ignite insight or lead to confusion and misunderstanding. Our society lacks English words for describing integral concepts related to yoga. Here's a short list from a long list I maintain. Think of it as your word/asana collection instead of stamps or birding list. Try them on, play with using them in different settings, or tweak them to get your point across. Having the flexibility to choose words wisely is a great hobby and skill to develop.

Mindsight: The capacity to cultivate integration, empathy, and insight. Contrasted with physical sight: Habitual visual focus on things outside ourselves. How do you train your mindsight (Siegel 2017)?

A working definition of mind: Mind is embodied and relational, a self-organizing emergent process that regulates the flow of energy and information both within and between humans (Siegel 2017, pp.56–57). Consistent and familiar to modern science. How about for non-professional audiences? Harder, isn't it? But can you feel how the word choice breaks down the misconception of mind as being the brain, or limited to within me?

Energy: Often associated these days with New Ageisms, Siegel corrected early on: "Is this some metaphysical proposal of energy patterns that are hard to grasp? Well, not really. Energy is a scientific concept, a process that exists in the physical world, not beyond it—it is not meta-physical" (2017, p.55) and then defined energy by a standard physics definition as the potential to do work. Sense how proper word choice dispels all the silliness or preconceptions that might otherwise cloud or block communication using the word energy?

Felt texture: Both word choice and metaphor. The words refer to our experience when we hold in awareness energy and information flow (Siegel 2017). Our subjective experience that emerges from this flow of time is a feature of the flow, but not the same as it. Often that energy and information flow happens without awareness and therefore we don't experience the felt texture. Once attention is redirected to sensing the tingles, prickles, current, pulsing of texture it is felt again. Seems safer to a larger audience than "feel the prana or chakra," at least to me.

Attunement: The focus of attention on the internal world; both personal and interpersonal between us and others. What happens to the tune without attention both personally and interpersonally? Not very good music or harmony, right? Or a bad tune (Siegel 2017, p.227).

To "feel felt" and "mWe": Feeling felt describes a phenomenon reported by clients as beneficial and indicative of a good therapeutic session. Because it includes personal and interpersonal, neither me or we is sufficient, so Siegel blended them as mWe to communicate that experience for which we had no good word (2017). MWe is to integrate our identity, to embrace not only the differentiated *me* with its personal in-group, and the differentiated broader *we* as a wider relational self, but also have both, together, that we can call this mWe (2017, p.322). As a plural verb rather than a singular noun, we are forever unfolding in how mWe takes in and receives, observes and narrates, sends out and connects, as we become not merely a set of neural responses to stimuli, but a fully embodied part of the deeply interconnected relational world in which we are embedded (p.325). Whoa. But can you sense how it begins to offer communication more effectively than, "We are all one"? And having the new word helps us sense that experience, broadening our awareness for a principle grounded in yoga.

"This journey we are on, exploring the inner and inter, diving into subjective seas and scientific concepts, complex systems and self-organization" and "But the self is not bound by skull or skin. The mind, and the self that comes from it, is embodied, yes, but is also fully relational. Honoring the personal self of me and the interconnected self of we, we link these two with the integrated self of MWe" (Siegel 2017, p.325). Just appreciate how the choice of words brings to life what we have all experienced, but not been able to express. Again, these are just examples from Dr. Siegel. Now start collecting the ones that work for you, and if you need be, create some new ones.

Translation of Old to New

As you read or attend workshops, discover new ways people are saying old things. There's really nothing new, just ways of saying the same things in the current language of the day. Here are two examples to get you started:

Extended mind: Partial description of mind not limited to the individual. Research includes cognition as: embodied, embedded, extended, situated, and emergent. Who knew there were so many flavors to choose from? Well, if you go back to classic texts on mind, seems there were a fair number of traditions, but we need to update from Sanskrit or the Pali, and so on. Or just read people like Thompson and Stapleton (2009) to build your modern vocabulary.

The gunas: Siegel (2017) describes how complex systems function across time with elements of rigidity (tamas?), chaos (rajas?), and integration (sattva?) all intermingling and all present in varying degrees from supportive to counterproductive. Sounds like a twenty-first-century description of the gunas, perhaps? Later he discusses how that model applies to trauma, as rigidity in people's lives makes life predictable, boring, without vitality, contrasted with chaos where life can be "explosive, unpredictable and filled with distressing intrusions of emotion, memory, or thought" (p.76). Can you find the gunas explanation, then, when he discusses posttraumatic stress disorder (PTSD) as being a life full of both chaos/rajas (intrusive bodily sensations, images, emotions, memories) and rigidity/tamas (avoidance behaviors, numbing, amnesia) (p.77)? Isn't this fun and fascinating? Or am I an even bigger nerd than I feared?

Memory Aides (Acronyms, Memes, etc.)

Another collection to start if you haven't already, is memory aides. Did you know there's a RAT in Parkinson's disease? From my 1981 physical therapy classes, Rigidity, Ataxia, and Tremor. Still got it. Structures across the front of your elbow crease, outside to inside? TAN. Tendon,

Artery, and Nerve. Here are few yoga-related examples to get you started and to help your students remember important principles.

- Can't heal what you don't feel (Author unknown).

- It isn't how far you go, but how you go far that matters (Author unknown).

- Integration is a direction, not a destination (Siegel 2017).

- Optimum self-organization is FACES: Flexibility, Adaptability, Coherence (having resilience), Energy, Stability (Siegel 2017).

- "Between and within us: A concise way of stating the flow of energy and information as mind" (Siegel 2017, p.70).

- "PART: Presence, Attunement, Resonance, and Trust. Qualities that if we bring into our teaching prime for the experience of 'felt mind' or being felt in the relationship" (Siegel 2017, p.167).

- "COHERENCE: Connected, Open, Harmonious, Engaged, Receptive, Emergent, Noetic, Compassionate, and Empathic. Siegel's definition of mental health" (Siegel 2017, p.89).

- "Kindness and compassion are integration made visible" (Siegel 2017, p.330).

- "Humankind: Can we be both?" Chapter title from Siegel (2017). Brilliant juxtaposition and question from a word we have all heard many times before.

What are some of your favorites?

Use a Picture

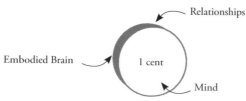

Aspects of One Reality

I created this picture from Siegel's (2017) description of how reality is like a coin, composed of mind, relationships, and embodied brain. Remove any one of the three aspects and reality is incomprehensible. A modern attempt at describing a triune concept (3 in 1), not far from St. Patrick's alleged use of the shamrock to describe the Trinity of Christianity.

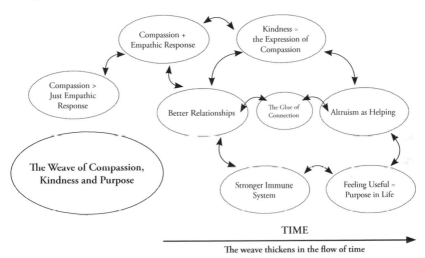

TIME

The weave thickens in the flow of time

Compassion Model

Here's my attempt to illustrate Jinpa's description of compassion (2015, pp.12, 16, 19).

In the upper left, "compassion is a more empowered state and more than an empathic response to the situation" (p.12). Jinpa noted that kindness is the expression of that compassion through helping, a basic form of altruism, shown on the far right. The emergence of compassion is what makes it possible for our empathic reaction to manifest in kindness. He also reflected that "the most compelling thing about compassion and kindness is how they bring purpose to our life. There is nothing like the feeling of being useful" (p.16). Kindness, he wrote, acts like glue to keep connections with our loved ones strong, thereby protecting us against the "fissures or breaks" (p.19) that disagreements and emotional distance may cause. Another anchoring thread is that, when compassion is demonstrated, it contributes to better relationships. Researchers have found that better social connection strengthens our immune systems. The common thread of kindness can be visualized as a key factor in forming and maintaining social connection, helping relationships, purpose/identity, and keeping our immune system healthy. Does the illustration help "see" or understand the words he offered? There will be several practices to reinforce this principle. Just trying to draw the rough sketch now anchors the relationships in my memory. Try it yourself.

Metaphor

We *use* metaphors (oops, there's one) to communicate reality to one another. They *work* (another one) but, as representations, *contain* error and limitations as well. (You can look inside a metaphor and see errors?) Am I making my point? So as with all our definitions, we need to become aware of the inherent vrittis that metaphors can create. The *key* (for what lock?) is that we hold and use them with humility and the proper sense of uncertainty.

Moseley and Butler's *Explain Pain Supercharged* (2017) has an entire chapter dedicated to metaphor and refer to metaphors throughout the book. The authors note that "pain is enemy" is our most dominant metaphor around pain. The images used in both describing pain and treating it convey mental pictures of weaponry and damage to include: fight pain, shooting or stabbing pain, and attack of pain, as well as painkillers, defeat pain, win the battle with pain, and so on. At the very least these enemy metaphors are not very yogic, but, as the book brilliantly describes, not at all helpful from the pain science perspective for supporting individuals with chronic pain, as we will visit later in this book. They argue the adoption of "pain as protector" with secondary metaphor possibilities such as "sore but safe and pain is a gift" (p.145). Can you feel or see the difference? Powerful, those metaphors (see their little buffed muscles?).

Mindsight is a metaphor. Siegel's (2017) *looking* inward at the aspects of mind. We have no good words for this process. Notice how the metaphor suggests a concept we teach. And another Siegelian metaphor: "we'd now say that the mind is fully embodied, not just *enskulled*" (p.46) and later, not just *enskinned* but between. Can you feel those two metaphors? Pictures that communicate old understandings and set up the *landscape* for new understanding.

And one more from Siegel (2017): "With presence as our portal for integration, kindness for the mind is as natural as breathing for the body" (p.330). Peering through the *portal* of presence, can you sense the integrated mind *breathing* kindness? What pictures does that metaphor evoke for you? Related is "The mind is the *heart* of being human" (p.212).

Storyteller in Chief

Finally, Siegel describes how stories bind us to each other, helping us make sense of our experiences, and allow us to learn from each other, thereby enhancing our relational lives (2017). For instance, when describing integration as the basis of health he shares a personal story about his experience of integration, "Now we can see this (integration) as the natural push of self-organization to pull me out of the states of rigidity and chaos, the two states that complexity theory tells us systems enter when they are not optimizing self-organization" (p.83). As a reader I was connected to his story, and had images to both organize and remember the abstract concepts of rigidity, chaos, and complexity theory.

We are, after all, just a group species of primates that have huddled around campfires telling stories and creating art to illustrate important aspects of being human. That's what you do either in private or group classes too. The language we select, the arc of the story we employ (the arc works for us, right?), and the way we hold a space to listen to the other's story are what we do. If you have never specifically studied the art of storytelling, I strongly encourage you to read a bit and tweak your storytelling asana. Just some small cues can make a big change in your ability to create relief from suffering. This is just the first time storytelling will be highlighted. More tales ahead.

I just used several examples of storytelling related to pain and mind as those are the focus of this book. I hope this next section describing the implications of our new understanding of yoga and yoga therapy on addressing pain will be a worthy example. You tell me.

A Painful Pause

Pain has its own chapter ahead. We will destroy your understanding of pain in Chapter 4, but for now consider some of these musings on the topic. As you know, pain is woven into all human experience, and so too, throughout this entire book. My Minnesota vignette is one thread.

Each chapter will also have pain and suffering sections as seen through that chapter's respective focus. In this chapter describing the implications of our new yoga understanding I share some basic pain concepts as they can be situated differently than the way they are traditionally presented in yoga. In Chapter 3 on wisdom, we will situate pain in a broader, historical context with other wisdom traditions. Given that, here's a pain appetizer.

Pain and suffering are what drove many of us to yoga. Somewhere along the way in our experience we probably experienced some relief and noted we were healthier and more comfortable from our practice. Our students also give us similar feedback which sustains us as providers of the teachings. It behooves us then to reflect on how we define pain and suffering, and to be able to describe how yoga is related to our definitions. No small task and no simple answers of course. Hence just this initial taste, as we will entertain pain throughout the rest of the book.

Patanjali Yoga Sutra 2.16 is often cited as a starting point. *Heyam-Dukham-Anagatam*: "The pain that is yet to come is to be avoided." Various translations use "may" be avoided, suggesting a purpose for yoga practice. Duhkah (suffering) is also how Life is described in the First Noble Truth of Buddhism, "Life is suffering." A third common reference are the kleshas noted in Patanjali's Yoga Sutra. Kleshas are listed as the five causes of afflictions, to include: Avidyâ "ignorance," asmitâ "I-am-ness," raga "attachment," dvesha "aversion," and abhinivesha "the will to live" (Feuerstein 1998). I am presuming these are all familiar to yoga professionals, and, if they are not, I encourage you to do further research.

For our purposes in this chapter, I want to highlight that these references point to a wide-ranging definition of pain and suffering beyond what could be a "clod" of limiting pain to individual physical and mental afflictions. Rather, the list is broad to include sorrow, disappointments, injustice, betrayal, racism, loneliness, loss, trauma-related disorder, and so forth. This broad net suggests we do not fall into the trap of presuming the reported complaint's location (our own or the student's) is also the source of the suffering. That horrendous headache or nagging back pain is better understood to be intimately related to the person's lived experience, including their BME. Unlike our modern mechanistic bias that the hip is "out," text neck, and so on, the first cause may be a psychospiritual misperception and hence the need for a psychospiritual practice such as yoga to discover the source of suffering.

Equally perplexing is the paradox around pain and suffering. A paradox being two statements that contradict one another, but are both true. We will spend some time with paradox in the wisdom chapter coming up, but consider this paradox: Pain and suffering is personal. Pain and suffering isn't personal, but shared. Say what? This isn't new, in fact it is how classical teachings have treated the topic. Our new understanding around yoga and yoga therapy makes addressing the paradox just more acute. The implications arise from the heart of our definitions. Your student's suffering isn't theirs alone, but also yours. And yours is also theirs. When the two of you work to alleviate or ease present or future suffering, it is for both of you and the rest of us. The more difficult side of this paradox is that when we seek to understand the source, there isn't one, but multiple and complex relationships to address at many levels. Oh no! Sense the burden of responsibility? The enormity of the task? Feel the objections rising up? It's just a backache. True. And isn't. Your back aches after gardening all weekend. You gardened all weekend because your schedule is so overcommitted it's the only time you had to garden. You are overcommitted why? Why couldn't you ask for help? Why didn't you stop when your body signaled fatigue? Why do you have to grow your own clean vegetables instead of being able to buy quality produce locally? See it? Feel it? Being able to rest in the tension of this and many other paradoxes is our practice. While resting in them, can we gain insights that weren't immediately apparent? What are spiritual issues here? There we go again, down the slide into complexity and relationships. We will come back to technique.

For now, at this point in the book, just keep in mind our "clod" of wanting to find *the* source of pain, and break that clod up by appreciating that there are probably numerous influences that need to be discovered. In fact, when we get to the pain chapter, we'll explore in detail how defining pain is every bit as slippery as defining yoga. Just know our job as yoga professionals is to create the safe environment for inquiry by the student to empower them to the create new responses, free of their former reactive patterns of behavior. And we can't know what their response should be, because we have not lived their experiences in their body. In this humility of unknowing and uncertainty, it's my responsibility to offer you a process of new perspectives and practical guidance. Unlike so many pain books, we won't have a recipe though, but rather will be more like finely trained chefs able to imagine and marry whatever ingredients present themselves to us. And unlike the passive viewers of the TV chefs who can't cook any better having watched the show, our students will be empowered to create feasts from their unique circumstance now and in the future because of their yoga process.

Now that we've whetted our appetite for pain and suffering, let's browse the remaining buffet of additional implications related to our new understanding of yoga and yoga therapy.

Spiritual Smorgasbord

Given that we are purveyors of a psychospiritual practice, not just glorified exercise instructors, how do we act like it? This is a unique period of human spirituality. Never before have humans had access to nearly every spiritual practice on the planet. What a treasure that's available to us, with our yoga being only one of many practices. In the next chapter we delve much deeper into this idea and where we fit in the traditions. What I want to address here is how do we restore our, and our students', spiritual practice through yoga? Do we have the skills to create a discovery of how, as a psychospiritual practice, yoga can support any familial spiritual tradition, negating the need to cast out tradition completely, and instead appreciate the tradition as related, not separate from their present life?

Paraphrasing Rohr (2013, p.137) we might consider yoga as the microcosm of the macrocosm or what Shakespeare would call "the play within the play." What's taking place within our small self, individualistic reality is also being acted out in the larger world stage. Therefore, no matter the individual's history, our individual suffering as we discussed in the last section is everyone's suffering. We've just told different stories across time trying to make meaning from our cultural and personal experience. Our role now as teachers is to forever hold together (yoke?) matter and spirit, divine and human, and to say they always have been one, but you, the student, just don't know it yet or have forgotten. Said with yoga language, Ishvara is going to hold matter and spirit together in front of their face until they do experience it. Maintaining a split or othering of their prior experiences doesn't allow that re-cognition (re-thinking about).

There's been in my experience a tendency for yoga to attract disaffected practitioners of religious traditions. What's your experience been? How do you address that disaffection? I've heard and read where the Dalai Lama advocates people return to their faith of origin. Matthew Fox (2004a) wrote *Many Wells, One River*, a compendium of our universal drive to realize the yoga of reality with whatever concept of divine and secular is being utilized. Celtic poet and former Catholic priest John O'Donohue (2017) said:

> To have access to a religious tradition is a huge, strengthening, critical resource, which keeps you wide awake and makes you ask yourself the hard questions. I've always thought that tradition is to the community what memory is to the individual. And if you lose your memory, and you wake up in the morning, you don't know where you are, who you are, what ground you're standing on. And if you lose your tradition, it's the same thing.

He acknowledged, as we know, that each tradition has its dark zones of sometimes complete horror. But they all as human institutions also have zones of great light and immense "wells of refreshment and healing." I agree with his assertion that it is important for somebody who wants to have a mature, adult, open-ended, good-hearted, critical spiritual practice, to conduct the "most vigorous and relentless conversation that you can with your own tradition" (O'Donohue 2017). Failure to do so results in a separation within one's life, and a doorway to suffering. I'm advocating the conversation, not necessarily having to return. Let's consider a bit more context as to why this is my suggestion.

As a teaser for the next chapter, know that yoga is part of the perennial tradition defined by Aldous Huxley in his book *The Perennial Philosophy* (2004). Huxley felt that this teaching was ageless and universal, that: (1) there is a Divine Reality substantial to the world of things; (2) there is an inner compatibility and coherence between humans and the Divine; and (3) the goal of human existence is quite simply union with that Reality. Wow, there's some *word choice*. He equates love of others, love of self, and love of God throughout his teaching. This unitive/yoga or non-dual consciousness understands such a teaching and such a philosophy.

Otherwise the dualistic mind just takes sides and stands isolated on one side or the other. Either God is great (too much religion), or humans and creation are great in and of themselves and by themselves (which can't be logically sustained), leaving the real synthesis that both are great (Rohr 2013). So, without that "relentless and vigorous conversation," we remain in separation.

Rohr (2013) stated that transformation is blocked when the separate self is the problem, to include our historical spiritual practice. He writes, "Whereas most religion and most people make the shadow self the problem. This leads to denying, pretending, and projecting instead of real transformation into the Divine" (2013, p.251). Exploring and knowing how both the bright and dark sides of our experience inform our present BME is crucial for transformation, to include easing suffering.

Am I suggesting we or our students will come to a certainty about our relationship with that former practice? Quite the opposite. An engagement of this type of yogic reflection and discernment will lead to a deep sense of humility. In the Christian tradition that state is referred to as "The brilliant cloud of unknowing." Unless we or our students have made it to enlightenment, we need to get comfortable with the fact that the beauty of what we aren't conscious about is that our unconscious is still an aspect of us that knows a great deal, whether personal or collective. Our unconscious always knows that it does not know, cannot say, dare not try to prove or assert too strongly, because what it does know is that there is always more and the humility to know all words will fall short. Rats, more uncertainty. As a yogi we are the person who agrees to live in that unique kind of light and dark. The paradox, of course, is that it does not feel like much brightness at all, but more like what others call "learned ignorance." Apparently, we need a strong tolerance for ambiguity, an ability to allow, forgive, and contain a certain degree of anxiety, and a willingness to not know and not even need to know. This is how we can allow and encounter mystery. Sorry if that isn't very satisfying, but it does carry forward the theme we've been working on so far.

This humility then can lead us to the silence within that Cloud of Unknowing. Meister Eckhart said, "Nothing in all creation is so like God as silence." And again, "The best and noblest of all that one can come to in this life is to be silent and let God work and let God speak"…this place of silence, which Eckhart calls "the doorway of God's house" (Fox 2016, p.66). Sounds pretty yogic for a German priest at the turn of the fourteenth century. The practice of silence is the entry way into creativity and makes up some of our first practices in the practice chapter. Not surprisingly, as far as pain and suffering are concerned, none of us go into our spiritual maturity completely of our own accord, or by a totally free choice. We are led by Mystery, which religious people rightly call grace (Rohr 2011). Might this be the doorway or threshold that the pain and suffering being addressed invites us to step through and transform? More loss of control and certainty, but *certainly* a recurrent theme across human history?

As we consider our religious history as a part of our spiritual practice and how it relates to our yoga now, it helps me to remember the origin of the word religion. Rohr writes, "this is what makes something inherently religious: whatever reconnects (re-ligio: tie together again) our parts to the Whole is an experience of God, whether we call it that or not" (Rohr 2011, p.xxxiv). To not address this important part of each of our BME is to fall short of relieving future suffering, even though I'm not sure there's an asana to do it.

As we'll explore in Chapter 3, my concern is that if we do not find that unitive yoga within ourselves and our past, we'll miss our complex and inexplicable caring for each other as well. Can there be healing to life's inconsistencies and contradictions with such a divide in our own experience? When done right, Rohr (2011, p.59) encourages us that, "Religion, with all of its faults, is always about getting one back and down into a unified field, where we started anyway." Hey, we made it to beginner's mind. Good work. Now, having sewed up this awkward religion conversation, is there a place for a psychospiritual practice in healthcare too? Perish the thought!

Yoga Therapy Should Be Everywhere in Healthcare

Sat Bir Khalsa, PhD, the driving force behind the research section of IAYT for the past decade and co-editor of its PubMed indexed journal, gave an important plenary address at the association's 2017 symposium. The talk was titled "The Road to Incorporating Yoga Therapy into Healthcare." He captured many important implications about the type of yoga therapy we are defining as a psychospiritual practice. I'll summarize his findings here for us. A fine complement to this summary are the perspective pieces, one of which I wrote with Dr. Timothy McCall, MD, on the current state of how yoga therapy is presently being delivered in the USA and worldwide in the 2017 issue of the journal (Taylor and McCall 2017).

Khalsa began his lecture by stating the road into systems in our culture is research evidence, to sway administrations and boards of directors of states, schools, and health-related organizations. He then offered that, rather than try win a comparison contest with already offered modalities, all of which are reactive (headache, back pain, depression, etc.), there is an even wider road available if we zoom our collective lens out further.

That road is the epidemic of non-communicable diseases (NCDs). These NCDs are the result of lifestyle and dysfunctional behavior, to include stress, diet, and sedentary habits. Combined, they are the leading cause of death (obesity, diabetes, heart disease, etc.). He then shared the research around the three leading factors and how current healthcare had no strategy for addressing any of them, while there is evidence yoga can change these behaviors. Those factors were: (1) Stress: There is no non-pharmacological strategy; (2) Awareness: No strategy for enhancing awareness physically or psychologically; and (3) Patient worldview: No strategy to address the rat race, materially oriented culture that requires a change in life purpose and meaning toward a unitive consciousness/spirituality for greater flow. Note all three are psychospiritual issues.

Our road then requires we educate and demonstrate how yoga is far more than a physical practice of exercise. The new yoga we've defined teaches mindbody skills and is multimodal in orientation. I'm sharing the language that is key that we adopt. Good news, there's a big problem standard healthcare cannot address. There's more good news: Yoga can, and we have the evidence and more on the way.

But the big insight was the research he shared that exists on how yoga alters spiritual perspectives and the documented transcendence that practice brings. Not in some religious sense, but in literally expanding the awareness of relationships. Yoga allows students to sense their body, how it is affected by movement, diet, and social circumstances. That new awareness, once established, has been demonstrated to change future behaviors toward functional healthy choices around activity, diet, stress, and social environmental factors. And this transcendence can happen in a very brief period of time. Transcendence as a word can be misunderstood, so let me be clear in this instance I'm using it not as meaning a rugged independence ruling over everything else, but rather as one remembering that we are bound up in the web of life. This transcendence means that participants move from an external "something outside me controls my health" toward a power within and the ability to overcome the false transcendence hierarchy as conceived by modern healthcare, where we have been taught to look up to healthcare for our health.

As the sincere Harvard scientist he is, he then shared the exponential increase in studies, many now random control trials (the highest form), and with it, the same growth in yoga-related research journals. Most of the new studies are focused on the biggest health challenges of mental health, cardiovascular health, and respiratory disease. He finished with a charge for us to build efficacy (it works) and cost effectiveness (money spent returns more benefit than it costs). Research shows the study participants believes yoga increases their health. Now we need to create delivery systems to teach that increased self-awareness avoids bad health behaviors. We are back to self-ethics and self-identity, it seems.

Bringing the implications Dr. Khalsa shared into practice will require a deeper understanding of many systems-related issues and structures, as well as creativity, because today's circumstances haven't existed before. For that reason, I keep writing and you keep reading.

Change the World off the Mat

We know yoga works. We also know what has been done with limited effectiveness with yoga thus far in our modern culture. Now is not the time to retreat to our zafu and presume change will happen. I'm not suggesting we abandon meditation, but I do worry that in our changing world very often yoga becomes a retreat from the larger world for both professionals and students. It's that old familiar trap of asmitâ and I do yoga for me. The definition of yoga and yoga therapy recognizes the intertwined relationship between the small self, small mind, individual worldview, and the reality of the larger Self, shared mind, and lived experience of BME of all of us. Uncomfortable asana isn't just some posture on the mat, but how we engage in an embodied way with our community. Yoga is not a practice of disengagement from that responsibility, but a sharpening acuteness of awareness of how important it is we create a best possible future for everyone. What are the implications for your local practice?

One implication is to ask: Does your personal practice lead to the healthy behaviors Dr. Khalsa outlined in the section above? Have you become more engaged or less engaged in your relationship with your local community and its needs? Have you gotten comfortable in your practice that pays the bills and lets you spend time with nice people? What hard edge have you played with becoming more active in your community? All of these things we won't avoid in Chapter 7 on practices.

Additionally, when's the last time you scrutinized your business model, marketing plan, and spending investment habits? Are they in line with your yoga ethics? That ethical self-review? If it has been a while and, without the context of this new understanding, then the next section is a must read and do.

There's a misperception that our yoga practice is all about love and acceptance. Baloney. While you are scrutinizing, did you find some areas you or your business are holding back from right action? We can respond strongly, but often avoid it due to all manner of habits and patterns. Sometimes we need to rise up, declare our truth, march, protest, do whatever is necessary to protect our life and the lives of others. This requires skill and strategy to be effective and non-harming. Exemplars in the past have rallied others, recruited the legal system, engaged in civil disobedience, negotiated, formed alliances, and artfully employed money, power, shame, speeches, and politics to participate in right action. Look again, are you assuming the full power available to you or have you settled for something less? I know too often I settle. This is our bigger practice.

Related, but scaled down a bit, how are you building a road into making your community healthier without sacrificing your health? Doing the same old tired pattern of behaviors your colleagues are practicing? How's your research literacy? Is your business culturally competent and marketed to engage the market where they are or just the 5–10 percent of early adapters that will try anything? Are you visible in the community and collaborating with others to make changes in behavioral health?

Do others seek you out for all those resources Dr. Khalsa described? If not, how can they discover that you exist? So much to do. Not to worry. There's much to explore yet and many simple, practical guidelines ahead. One bit at a time. Let's relax and talk about money next!

Moola Toning Exercises

Money, what's that got to do with the last chapter? A great deal it turns out. The historical deconstructionists I mentioned do an excellent job of describing how yogins in the past were sustained and funded. Particularly interesting is to read how the late nineteenth and early twentieth-century yogis who traveled made their way through foreign cultures. Had they not been reasonably adept, you wouldn't be reading this book.

As a generalization, in my experience the yoga community is averse to talking about money and typically bad at managing money. I have consulted with yoga businesses, sat on boards of directors, and taught the business section of IAYT for several years. There are entire books that have been written on the topic, to include "spiritual" money management of good and poor quality. If you are bad at it, read some or get a qualified business coach. My friend and colleague Matthew Sanford has put it simply, "Consciousness follows money." Pair that with the accurate proverb of "The *love* of money is the root of all evil" (money isn't evil). An additional factor is that in our society of selling everything. Nora Bateson (2017, p.109) reasons, "We can sell off everything for money because it allows us to not see the relationships that exist once something is monetized." Therefore, we need to exercise caution and awareness around money at a much deeper level than most of us have been trained to do in our culture. Another instance where ignorance isn't bliss.

These considerations imply that in order for you to fulfill your dharma as a yoga therapist, and your student(s) to fulfill their dharma, the skills of financial competence are essential asana to practice. Bad financial alignment, no good flow of consciousness. There's no excuse. Money is a form of prana. Manage/regulate it well. Poor management is himsâ (harming) and avoidance is a klesha. Get over it and master the skills so you can deliver your dharma to ease both your and your student's suffering. Not a long section of this book, but without it, my yogic powers see suffering in your future.

Hamstring Stretching [sic] for Organizations

The implications of the new ways of defining mind earlier in this chapter suggest great possibilities for yoga therapy being used to support dysfunctional, suffering organizations and institutions. I have written an entire textbook chapter on this topic, but let me see if I can share the highlights and make you hungry for more (Taylor 2015a). Can you hold what we discussed about mind being interpersonal as well as intrapersonal? And the extended consciousness studies that takes mind beyond the skull and the skin of the individual? Couple that with the paradox of pain and suffering being both personal and not. Now add all of that to the asmitâ of both the student and you the yoga professional, misperceiving you are both separate and therefore the owners/fixers of suffering. Now you have your hands full. Let's try to unload some of all that.

Consider these observations:

- The individual lived experience includes our relationships within our environment.

- The individual human is no longer the most complex living entity on the planet. That's multinational corporations (Senge *et al.* 2004).

- Those corporations are composed of individuals.

- Efforts to introduce yoga and mindfulness into organizations via what I call "lunchroom yoga" fail to address the instabilities of the mind of the organization.

- Too often those programs are used solely to increase productivity and lower costs, not address the culture and other environmental relationships causing suffering.

- The most effective way to change large systems is through the personal practice of the individuals in a way that empowers them to make change in structure and policy (Senge *et al.* 2004).

- The emerging science of organizational development and change utilizes very yoga-like activities to foster change and innovation (Scharmer 2007).

- The observation that the "bio-logic," or pattern of organization, of a simple cell is the same as that of an entire social structure is not trivial. It suggests a fundamental unity of life, and hence we also the need to study and understand all living structures from such a unifying perspective (Capra and Luisi 2016).

- Business is alive with the buzzwords of resilience, social creativity, transformational learning, and sustainability. These are yoga outcomes that are more appealing than just stress management. Use them.

- Now is the time to acknowledge the failures of standard economic theory and the narrowness of market fundamentalism. The times demand a revolution in economic thought. Human needs are finite, but human greed is not, economic growth can usually be maintained through artificial creation of needs by means of advertising. How does this mindset change in yoga?

- However, you might not want to tell the leadership that organizational yoga is not just keeping the troops calm, but a powerful igniter of change that often includes Kali and Shiva-like destruction as part of the growth. Real yoga doesn't produce well-behaved automatons. As John O'Donohue (2017) said, "it's a dangerous thing to have a soul." Restoring the soul in a place of soulless work is very combustible.

- Organizational yoga therapy is embryonic right now. There are no prior models to consult or mimic. We need to create it.

The implication of this section is that we yoga professionals need to become the vanguard of bringing organizational yoga therapy to institutions. To do so will require that we quicken the pace of our own evolution, broadening our context to match our culture, and acquiring the skills needed to create new programming. The benefits for us as individuals, institutions, and the planetary community are so needed right now.

The same fervor that fueled our early asana and classical yoga study now needs to be applied toward becoming competent to discover, create, and deliver practices that incorporate innovative systems to deliver for organizations in ways that we can't even imagine today. How do we do this? Within the complexity of our circumstance lies the simplicity of the sutras and modern day organizational change: we sustain a personal daily practice. And we keep reading this book to learn more about wisdom, pain, and fostering that need creativity. Yoga as a part of the wisdom traditions will be key in navigating your way toward your intentions.

I hope we have disassembled and started to reassemble a new framework of understanding around yoga. We widened the lens of implications based on this understanding beyond the studio or clinic perspective. Having this new perspective has tilled the soil of our now not so hard-packed understanding for appreciating the broader place yoga has in the wisdom traditions as explored in the next chapter. Possibly you can sense the "movement" of assimilation and intuiting new ideas and insights percolating up around you and your practice? Ideally you might be at peace with less knowing and fresh questioning. Could that be wisdom on the horizon?

3

. . .

Wisdom: That's You

MINNESOTA ADVENTURE

Twenty-two years later, I can appreciate the rare bit of counsel my dad had shared with me around that time. Before that trip I'd described to him my ambitions to build this, create that, and develop many other projects to which he replied to the effect, "Old Father So & So (sorry, dad, I don't remember who) said that young men dream big dreams, old men appreciate small things done well." The quote has shades of Mother Theresa or Teresa of Avila, but nonetheless within my botched recollection there rings a certain wisdom. To my reckoning today, being in my mid-30s as I was at the time might be considered the sophomore phase of adulthood [Greek *sophos* wise + *mōros* foolish]. At my physical and mental prime (aside from my back pain), I could work tirelessly for months on end and never had to refer to a patient record for details despite a crazy volume of patients. Couple that with listening to self-development cassettes driving to home health visits daily over my lunch hour and I pretty much knew it all. I thought.

And what about that paradox thing with pain being both personal and not that we discussed last chapter? Being flat on my back I was taking it all very personally. In fact, in retrospect, I think I had to because that was exactly where I was developmentally regarding wisdom. Had someone asked me then what wisdom was, I'd have answered something to the effect that it was someone that was very smart and had creative ideas. Not bad, but well short of describing wisdom. I am also quite sure I couldn't imagine, let alone describe how my present pain and suffering were anything but mine. Oh, maybe something about linking my suffering to Jesus's if I had been pressed for an answer based on my parochial education, but nothing I could feel or describe from a felt experience. So, lying there with that wise foolishness shattered in pieces, I was forced to consider not only how to "fix" my back, but also what was most important in life and what were my actual limits?

If this pain was going to continue, who and what could I become? And who knew the answers to my questions? I was burned out on the physical therapy gurus who I could now see saved their one nugget of gold for the last two hours of a course so I would stay the whole time. And the self-help crowd, why were their personal lives generally a mess, and how come there had to be so many of them if they had the answers I needed? I didn't realize it, but I was questioning authority for the first time.

Who has authority? Why? Where do I look for it? What was the function of my community of mentors, teachers, peers, and friends in determining that authority? Wisdom was knocking and I was forced to listen, lying there. What was keeping me from hearing? Was there value in my lived experience and could my body serve as a guide toward wisdom? How had being an "expert" in my community and work environment left me with so many blind spots or holes in my fabric of awareness and knowledge up in the woods? All my life I had given authority to something or someone outside myself. Was that a barrier preventing me from accessing wisdom without the fool part?

. . .

Not too wise, right? What concerns me today is seeing yoga professionals clamoring for the same solution to fix something either for themselves or their students. We've been very methodically taught to look outside ourselves for the authority or answer. That external focus coupled with a mechanistic understanding of pain is everywhere in the "yoga world," reflecting the same larger societal biases. In doing so, we have all steadily handed over authority and power to change, heal, and flourish as individuals and as societies. Little did I realize up there in the woods that I was about to undergo an accelerated course in wisdom training.

That training meant dismantling the mechanistic/parts worldview and redirecting my focus inward to assume my authority for my own life. My response-ability was going to be challenged. And how about you? What blind spots do you have? How do you fit into the wisdom traditions? (Spoiler alert: Being a yoga professional is no guarantee you are practicing wisdom.) What wisdom would you have imparted to me then if you were my teacher? Why that? Remember I was an "expert" with a deep knowledge base who longed to be right. While you consider those questions, allow me to share some of what I've picked up through a long, developmental process since I counted those nails holding the ceiling panels in my cabin ashram. Another easy chapter, this time all about wisdom in few pages.

Well here's a bit of irony. Early on in drafting the proposal for this book, I put together the title, "Teaching from the Wisdom of Pain," not fully appreciating the implication that I would then have to write about wisdom. The title changed, but the chapter is still here. Don't get me wrong, I love the topic. It's just that there are literally libraries packed with tomes addressing wisdom. How can I put a readable chapter together that both wisely addresses wisdom and has very practical outcomes for you as a reader? Here's my plan.

We begin by building a concise background on the history of wisdom and some current definitions. Next is a section addressing how wisdom has been treated in yoga both classically and currently, so there's some orientation in the sea of wisdom studies and the related challenges. From there we'll look at paradox and how wisdom points us toward the next chapter on pain as an emergent phenomenon. This section addresses paradigms, systems thinking, and tools required to grow in wisdom to include new vocabulary and qualities required to make such a shift in understanding. The chapter then concludes by addressing the question, "So what?" for a yoga professional. That section touches on current concerns over power and authority; reframing what becoming "wise" means in our hyper-media market; how yoga wisdom dovetails with our familial or cultural spiritual practices for broader integration; and a critical section situating us in the modern discussions dealing with integral relationships and culturally comfortable languaging of this yoga stuff we're trying to sell. Specific details are offered for the pain crisis, cautions for wisdom teachers, and vulnerabilities with the compassion "boom." This might be my favorite chapter and I suspect you won't find this information in any other yoga book. Without being woven into this fabric of wisdom, you are apt to float along and affect only superficial change.

Consider this bridging thought as we prepare to explore wisdom. Rohr (2013) stated that the opposite of rational (the cry of modern hubris) is not always irrational, but it can be transrational or bigger than the rational mind can process. Accepting the existence of this "too big to process rationally," as we approach wisdom, humility is in order in describing human challenges such as love, death, suffering, God, and infinity that are all transrational experiences. Hence these topics are also then in the domain of myth and what he calls "mature" religion that appreciates the existence of the transrational. With a humble spirit in the presence of human transrationality, may we have the capacity to keep us considering an open system and a larger horizon so that our soul, hearts, and mind do not close down inside some proud small, constricted space (Rohr 2011).

> The [use of] proof in the world has not provided the information that we need to see the complexity of the world we live in. We do not understand it. We make decisions that unfold into wild and unforeseen consequences. The proof was not enough. We needed the pattern. Art does not ask for proof; it directs us to look for pattern. (Bateson 2017, p.102)

Wisdom: Background and Some Definitions

Philosophers (lovers of wisdom) have been courting wisdom for centuries. What is wisdom? Who has it? And where does it come from? Those easy questions modern society studies in depth. Right! On the contrary, Rohr (2013) accurately points out that the irony of ego consciousness (small self) is that it always excludes and eliminates the unconscious—so our conscious is actually *not* conscious and therefore not wise. It seems the small self insists on knowing, on being certain, and it refuses all unknowing. Which is why you keep reading this uncertainty refrain each chapter. Most people who think they are fully conscious (read smart, enlightened, or wise) have a "big leaden manhole cover" over their unconscious (Rohr 2013, p.304). Their manhole covers give them control, but seldom compassion or wisdom. Gee, does this remind us of anything going on in our world today? Most major problems in our modern world reflect the need for wisdom. In fact, as the power of technology increases, so too does the need for wisdom, and it is no exaggeration to say that humankind is in a race between what Rohr (2013) calls "sagacity and catastrophe" (p.304). Once more, we need to surrender to uncertainty, so let's remove our manhole covers and spend time on this critical topic so rarely examined in modern society.

Before we begin, for the readers who want to go deep into wisdom research and delineations, I recommend Walsh (2015). It took some real wisdom to pull together what he did and he also offers a substantial bibliography.

The human experiences such as love, intelligence, creativity, yoga, pain, and wisdom are best appreciated as fuzzy constructions rather than sharply defined experiences. Wisdom has many forms, being complex, profound, and many varieties of subtypes. Further, it is closely related to other virtues such as benevolence and ethics. (There's that ethics again.) In addition to its profundity, there seems to be a developmental perspective, whereby certain stages of development are implied across an individual's lifetime, as well as along an evolutionary arc of the entire species. Within scientific inquiry, modern wisdom now also has diverse definitions with many recently designed measurement scales. Further complicating the attempt to define wisdom is the fact that the research has been generally limited to practical wisdom, overlooking the multiple varieties or subtypes of wisdom described over the ages (Walsh 2015).

A brief look at historical definitions includes the classical Greek division of sophia (theoretical) and phronesis (practical), both vague and used in various ways across the ages. Ray (2000) notes Buddhism has similar descriptions with prajna (transconceptual: refined and drawn from numerous disciplines) and upaya (practical wisdom). The Buddhists also distinguish between the mundane and supramundane wisdom, which also suggests a more accessible type of wisdom versus a more refined type requiring special skill levels. Walsh (2015) offers that we need to consider at least four subtypes of wisdom, one of which is the practical that responds to everyday life issues, while the remaining three—intuitive, conceptual, and transconceptual—are knowledge about life issues without direct applications (epistemic). These types will be described in more detail below.

The first subtype is practical wisdom, which is the wisdom displayed when everyday challenges arise and one makes a wise decision and acts accordingly. There is a real world problem that is solved wisely. Fairly solid stuff that one can "see" and appreciate. The second subtype, intuitive, we can't see and often results in wordless knowledge that the person having it cannot easily conceptualize or formulate; Sternberg (1998) considers such not easily explained knowledge as the core of wisdom. An example is when you ask someone how they knew what you appreciate as a bit of wisdom not involving a direct practical challenge and they shrug their shoulders and state, "I don't know, I can't explain it, I just knew." Intuitive wisdom is deep, accurate intuitive insight into oneself and the central existential issues of life (Walsh 2015). Contrast intuitive with a classic example of the third subtype, conceptual wisdom, depicted as the philosopher-sage. This is a person with both deep insight and an intellectually sophisticated understanding of life issues who can offer extended treatises describing the associations and relationships between concepts. They can essentially "see" the linkage of concepts and describe them, unlike the intuitive. So conceptual wisdom is deep, accurate, rich, and integrated understanding of oneself and the central existential issues of life (Walsh 2015).

Walsh also notes that contemplative disciplines and non-Western philosophies include the fourth subtype: transconceptual wisdom. Let's unpacked transconceptual wisdom. Contemplative disciplines are those traditions around the world, and often in conjunction with the major religions, that focus on mental training disciplines such as meditation, contemplation, and our yoga. This training also includes supportive practices such as ethics (yamas and niyamas), lifestyle (Ayurveda), community (sangha), instruction, reflection, and service to others (seva and karma) (Walsh 2015). These practices are said to cultivate psychological development and certain mental capacities such as mindfulness, focus, equanimity, and discernment. The practices are believed to nurture stages of progress through transpersonal stages of development, generating wholly new transformative deep insights into oneself and the nature of reality (Walsh 2015). Those insights create a unique transconceptual, transrational, or transcendental type of wisdom which reflects an apprehension of the fundamental nature of self and reality. Walsh documents these transconceptual wisdom traditions to include *prajna* (Buddhism), *jnana* (Hinduism), *ma'rifa* (Islam), *gnosis* (Christianity), and *zhi* (Neo-Confucianism). He describes a yoga example where a practitioner first listens to lessons (*sravana*), then reflects on teachings (*manana*) in order to develop conceptual understanding. Then the student meditates on them (*nididhyasana*) to develop a deeper intuitive apprehension, and hopefully enters a state of unmoving focus (*samadhi*) in which transconceptual wisdom (*jnana*) arises (Feuerstein 2014). Walsh (2015) suggested that, across time, wisdom can be described as a multifaceted, multidimensional, and multilevel skill, a function and makeup that varies across individuals, circumstance, schools, and tasks. More complexity and nuances. The patterns keep repeating for us.

When Walsh (2015) looked across many definitions he also identified a number of elements they had in common. Wisdom is said to have prosocial attitudes and include behaviors that are prosocial. Being wise also involves social decision making and pragmatic knowledge of life, and includes regular reflection and self-understanding. Wisdom further exhibits flexibility with increased value relativism and tolerance for diversity, as well as acceptance and effectively dealing with uncertainty and ambiguity. (Oh, that's why Taylor keeps harping on uncertainty.)

Seeing clearly is another common element, which is familiar to us as viveka, in jnana yoga, as one of the four principal practices of discernment (Feuerstein 1998). We visited this element in the first yoga chapter when we were discussing ethical review and the yamas/niyamas practices being a form of discriminative wisdom. Walsh also found numerous mentions of humor, spirituality, and openness to new experience used in defining wisdom. I hope this meandering discussion is providing a sense of the enormity of wisdom and how yoga is woven into the virtue.

Interestingly, the traditional claims of contemplative practices such as meditation and yoga that they enhance perceptual sensitivity and accuracy have recently received considerable experimental support that is beyond the scope of this book (Walsh 2015). Just know whereas long-term meditation may cultivate wisdom, it is possible that a single session prior to testing may activate wisdom, as do dialogue and certain visualizations in novices. Wisdom has the slippery property of becoming, being, developing and so much more, requiring us to...? How about, be tolerant of ambiguity and uncertainty?

The question of where wisdom is to be found has no simple answer. Some argue in people, others in cultural products and texts, while Walsh (2015) argues some resolution of the debate through the application of integral theory. That's the "wise" position I'm presenting in this chapter and I intend to demonstrate the reasons why I am and how that position supports the remainder of the book. The last thing we need is a *certain* definition of another complex topic! My intention is to offer a practical working definition that has real world benefits for you and those you serve. Even though we don't have certainty, we can resolve to use the definition "carefully and skillfully" (Walsh 2015, p.279).

Given this slippery fish, I am appreciative that Walsh went to great efforts to offer a working definition of wisdom based on his inquiry. I propose we adapt it given both the quality of the research that went in to it and because it meets my requirement that it be practical for our uses in this book.

Walsh's definition is:

Wisdom is deep accurate insight and understanding of oneself and the central existential issues of life, plus skillful benevolent responsiveness. (2015, p.282)

Let's break down this definition and lay some groundwork for both the pain and creativity chapters ahead. First we ought to ask, if we or our students aren't being wise, what is our usual mind state? If we apply the opposite words within the definition, it sounds quite familiar: superficial, inaccurate, little new insight with misunderstandings of both oneself and existential issues, all lacking benevolent responses. Ouch. Other descriptors include automatons, conventional, illusory, consensus trance, unreflective, and herd mentality (Walsh 2015). Not very flattering, but more common for me than I care to admit.

What I notice that changes and what we will practice throughout the remainder of the book is that when I move back toward expressing wisdom it includes the various subtypes. The more I apply and build conceptual understanding that informs and frames my insights, I can then link them together (integrate), and thereby create meaning around the issue at hand. Further contemplation seems to nurture the depth of my insight and understanding. Participating in study, reflection, dialogue, and meditation allows me to recognize and integrate more perspectives than just my unreflective habit of mind. This skill is said to increase developmentally across time and practice, with improved ability to recognize and integrate relationships between concepts and systems of concepts. That has been my experience and I have observed it in my students as well. Have you had a similar experience?

Is stringing together insights around concepts then wisdom and a way to become *deep and accurate*? Of course not. We have many forms of knowledge, to include the healthcare training model of hear one, see one, do one, and teach one. We are exposed to the concepts, we gain insight through observing the application of the concepts, we then gain practical, psychomotor knowledge through our embodiment of the concepts into action, and finally we have to present/teach to another using the knowledge gained from the previous steps as well the ongoing feedback in the teaching moment as we note the outcomes of the instruction. This understanding requires critical reflection at every stage. Our intended outcome is to produce intellectual rigor that is well processed, then integrated into our personal greater body of knowledge, and supported by enthusiastic conviction. Understanding then deepens through meditation and a regular process of internalizing our understanding until it becomes part of our basic mental landscape. It's a welcome relief when, at this final stage, the knowledge becomes effortless, integrated, and experiential. Jinpa (2015, p.203) summarizes the process succinctly, stating, "What was previously a deliberate cognitive understanding has transformed into an embodied spontaneous knowledge." For we yoga professionals, remembering teaching our first asana class and comparing that to offering a basic asana class now is a good example of this process.

Understanding of oneself of course is the focus of the niyamas in a yoga practice that moves beyond just asana instruction. This describes the gradual (and occasionally sudden) recognition of a deeper transpersonal Self and beginning to identify with that Self, rather than with the small self-representation (self-concept, self-image, ego). The small self was the conventional, former assumption of who and what I was, and this new recognition then enhances my self-understanding. This new understanding, as we mentioned in the yamas/niyamas discussion earlier, is said to be healing (making/realizing whole), but also freeing as both a liberation from the old unwise state and a form of enlightenment. The enlightenment, or "shining light on," describes a core realization of transconceptual wisdom that couldn't previously be grasped by the individual.

Self-knowledge is essential for sagacity, but so too is deep, accurate insight and understanding of *the central existential issues of life*. What are these issues? Existential issues are dilemmas that we all face, merely through our existence as human beings (Cooper 1990). In our age of superficial soundbites, little attention or reflection is given to questions about:

> the fundamental nature of identity and reality; the challenge of having an aging, mortal body; confronting suffering, sickness and death; living in personal and social relationships with others; constructing meaning and purpose in an apparently meaningless and mysterious world; selecting values and morals and then living up to them; and facing endless choices for which we alone are responsible. (Walsh 2015, p.285)

Can you sense the relative absence of this level of depth that is missing today?

Our drive for certainty and the dense marketing of the same false promises clouds the reality that life is always mysterious, our knowledge will never be complete, and, most disturbingly, the future is largely unpredictable. As Rohr (2013) noted earlier, no wonder we want to grab our manhole covers and avoid this wisdom work. It isn't for the faint-hearted. If we can't adopt the appropriate humility and acceptance of mystery, the result is a defensive ignorance which is the opposite of wisdom. We and our students face the personal challenge of deciding how to respond to these existential issues if we intend to teach from the wisdom of pain. No getting around it. Addressing abhinivesha (fear of death or dissolution) as a yogic klesha becomes imperative. That doesn't just mean calling that last asana in class "corpse pose" rather than "relaxation pose," but to approach these central issues on an ongoing basis. Without practical applications, we would all keep looping in conceptual wisdom without *skillful responsiveness*. Which is why practical wisdom is required.

The definition of practical wisdom is the skillful benevolent responsiveness to the central existential issues of life. Note the circularity within these definitions that reveals the integral nature of this work. It invites us to ask "What is skillful in this context?" The answer is actions that reduce suffering and enhance wellbeing including for oneself. We will see in Chapter 4 that to alleviate pain one needs to not only seek and see how to act benevolently, but also possesses the required skill to do so. There's an action required through an embodied engagement in one's environment that is dependent on knowing one's self *deeply and accurately* as one recognizes and lives in accord with both one's unique character and capacities and one's deeper universal nature. In the context of yoga teachings, we can say it as: Only by recognizing our svabhava (unique being) can we recognize our svadharma (unique life path) and the responses that are appropriate for us in each situation. Is that helpful in weaving wisdom to yoga to pain?

Our *accuracy* includes a humility in the face of uncertainty and mystery. Can you see some hints toward Arjuna's svadharma plight from the Bhagavad Gita in the following descriptions of the forms of wisdom? Wisdom requires an ability to discern appropriate responses. Check. That discerning requires not just a humility, but several forms. Of course, more complexity. Walsh (2015) describes three: (1) *Agential humility* that recognizes that there are some things we simply cannot change; (2) *Epistemic humility* that recognizes that we can never know all the factors involved in a situation; and (3) *Predictive humility* that recognizes the uncertainty of the final outcome and all the ramifications of our actions. Poor old Arjuna resisted pulling back that string on his bow, didn't he? But to deny these existential limits would be to live unwisely. The first two humilities reflect the core of St. Francis's Serenity prayer too, so no wonder I keep citing Fr. Rohr the Franciscan. Ultimately we can only get to both the right means and right ends by recognizing and responding appropriately to our human limitations. To not do so will cause us to be other than *benevolent*.

What is *benevolence* (*bene* = good, *velle* = wish)? We can describe it as the central intention of the wise, representing an outgrown egocentricity that is now deeply and altruistically concerned. There are ties to strong ethics, in our context through the yamas and niyamas. Wisdom, benevolence, and ethics are strongly overlapping and interdependent virtues. There's that weave of relationships again. Walsh (2015, p.285) summarizes, "The degree of wisdom is correlated with the scope and depth of benevolence." In addressing suffering and pain, we know wisdom is a function of development. Therefore, the wise will recognize and seek to optimize more mature kinds of wellbeing, whether that is us as professionals, or our students, in self-care. In other words, we should all intend to enhance not only general happiness, but also deeper kinds and sources of wellbeing contrasted with acting as mere symptom relievers. That intention then includes seeking greater growth and maturity in our own wisdom development. This focus on maturation reflects our yoga therapy definition of both process and direction, where we don't treat symptoms, but dive deep into the issues that are related to the suffering, knowing the importance of these levels of development for both the nature of wisdom and wisdom's expression through each of us.

In summary, wisdom and benevolence are linked. The wiser people are, the greater the number of people and creatures they seek to benefit, so the greater the time span they consider, and the deeper the kinds of benefit they seek to offer versus the less wise, who focus on fewer (or just one) people across a shorter time span. Prescribing superficial practice and chasing symptoms is to be avoided and will be critical for appreciating why we need to keep identifying and unlearning more before we tackle pain and creativity.

The Aspiration of Wisdom Yoga Practice

Here's a fascinating anchoring section back into our yoga profession. As we're learning, wisdom must be rooted in real world responsiveness or action of a benevolent nature. There's a tendency in considering wisdom and yoga philosophy to fall down rabbit holes of almost ethereal concept juggling and lose sight of solving problems. Yoga as a psychospiritual practice is quite ethereal in its aspiration to transcend or be liberated as a central aspiration. How might we balance such an aspiration with the demands of today's world? Asked another way, when sitting with a student in pain, do they truly care about achieving the transpersonal heights of maturity and wisdom, beyond the illusory, constructed nature of the usual self-sense to recognize their deep unity with others? Well, not if we say it that way.

We will be creating ways to say that better, but it's important to understand that classic unitive experiences are key to alleviating suffering and knowing how students can experience them and be situated within their context of the present circumstance is essential. We explore the importance of context setting and awareness later in this chapter. Right now, I want to highlight the question that as we do, as wisdom teachers, can we create learning experiences that bring forward something so aspirational and support the person in integrating that experience? Calling the experience by the historical names such as cosmic consciousness, numinous experience, peak experience, at-onement, holotropic, or transpersonal almost certainly won't get the job done for most students (Walsh and Shapiro 2006).

One of our tasks now is to create programming and processes that reveal how wisdom seeks to benevolently enhance the wellbeing of others (to include self) because it sees such actions as appropriate moral responses to suffering. Further, when we enhance wellbeing as an expression of enlightened self-interest it gives rise to a natural expression of our deep identity and interconnection with others. This, rising above and across (trans) concepts, is, of course, transconceptual wisdom. We've also hinted at the need for both emotional regulation and wisdom as being mutually facilitating to arrive at *deep and accurate insights*. Making the learning experience practical will be a matter of our integrating these many, but distinct virtues.

Can you feel your emotional response to all of this and the leaning toward "Well what's the solution?" I can. That attraction to certainty is our personal signal to return first to our own emotional regulation to remain in equanimity, which is defined as the ability to experience provocative stimuli fully and non-defensively without psychological disturbance. Walsh (2015) notes that equanimity has been little recognized in Western psychology except for occasional mention of related abilities such as "affect tolerance," "experience tolerance," and "emotional resilience." Historically this quest for imperturbability includes Sri Aurobindo (1993), one of India's greatest twentieth-century philosophers and sages, who described it as the characteristic temperament of the sage. Today we are faced without a certain solution to what these practices might be because we don't have the research literature to find our answers. I guess we're left with our own personal practice. Again. Let's then continue with some jnana practice evaluating some challenges to wisdom.

The Challenges of Wisdom

Blurry boundaries: Wisdom, like all virtues, is interdependent and complementary to other virtues and that can lead to some confusion of terms. Walsh (2015) noted that this lack of clear distinction reflects a repetitive problem in wisdom research. He explained that researchers recognize the need for diverse virtues to include non-attachment, emotional regulation, or compassion in order to fully explore wisdom. As wisdom teachers we too have the challenge of being able to describe the other qualities and virtues that complement wisdom. The dance of differentiating and integrating terms is an important one to be able to perform for students if we hope to achieve the *depth* of insights of wisdom. Finding that balance is what makes this chapter so difficult to craft. Hang in there, I promise the effort and attention is worthwhile.

Patience and tolerance: We need to keep in mind the challenge of the developmental nature of wisdom across time for ourselves and our larger community. Each new developmental stage gives us new capacities, insights, and understandings that were unavailable at earlier stages and quite literally, are not available to those of us at earlier stages. This is an old theme within yoga around the yarn, "When the student is ready, the teacher will arrive." In other words, until that time (development takes place across time), certain insights of the higher stages of development of wisdom won't be available to individuals. Without direct experience of these stages and states, the knowledge one has access to will be different in different states of consciousness. Walsh (2015, p.290) describes this as the "self-demanding capacity" of wisdom. Said another way, the challenge is we need to become wise in order to be wise, and to understand it fully we need to cultivate it in ourselves. This requires patience and tolerance toward ourselves and our students/community. A helpful example is as humans we need to develop through stages to understand the conservation of volume. You can show youngsters two different glasses of water, one a short, wide glass and another tall, skinny glass with the same amount of water and they'll insist the tall one has more water even as you pour that same amount back and forth between the two. They just don't "get it." Curiously, once they've developed the ability to conserve volume operationally, they understand immediately that it is the same volume and can't believe they ever couldn't understand it, even when shown video of their denial recorded earlier. Does that feel familiar for you around wisdom insights you've experienced as well? "Well of course I knew that!" Alas, not so much.

That self-care thing: The age-old challenge of balancing between the *oneself* and the others within the wisdom definition. We will address the importance of self-care later in this chapter in the compassion section. For now, how do we negotiate the challenge of selfishness versus too much sacrifice? Walsh calls it the benevolence of enlightened self-interest (2015, p.288). We need to seek a deep wellbeing, not just for ourselves, because that would be selfishness. But we must also not just be serving the wellbeing of others, which would be too much sacrifice. Where is the balance between self and others? Too much of either will create suffering. Selfishness as greed and jealousy creates conflicts and produces ill will with others, generating the opposite of recognizing our interdependence. By the same token, too much compassionate action might seem to be sacrifice but in the end generates burnout and resentment for oneself. Walsh admonishes us to continually seek balance and appreciate the "paradox of happiness," that is, by spending time and resources on others we can create more happiness than spending them on ourselves (Walsh 2011).

Desperately seeking simplicity: Nora Bateson (2017) beautifully addresses this challenge. Can all of this complexity of wisdom ever be applied in a practical way? She simply can't grasp how complexity can be understood as not practical. She wonders what one means by practical and what level of application they inquiring about? I share that confusion, but reading the above about the developmental nature of wisdom, I suspect I'm like the child with the glasses of water once I "get it" that only complexity is ultimately practical. This insight has helped me deal with my frustration, when so many other people I consider learned don't honor or acknowledge the complexity of human wellbeing. The drive for quick, simplistic thinking as solutions amounts to shortcuts that ultimately are misguided with unpleasant consequences. I had an editor write me once in reply to my concern about the limitations of presenting "regional interdependence" being too simplistic to understand orthopedic challenges. His reply in effect was that of course everything is connected to everything, but it wasn't practical! Bateson shares that same frustration when her work is described as ethereal and her students report being frustrated because the only "given" she offers is change. As you will read soon, she advocates that life is mutual learning. Life shifts and systems are in constant flux, and like it or not, that appears to be *reality* (one of those annoying central existential issues). She appreciates that reality sets up an:

> unspeakable beauty of those interdependencies that exactly matches the horror. The beauty lies in the ever-forming symmetries and asymmetries that evolve into unimaginable grace, and the horror in the sense that there is so much uncertainty and so little control. (2017, p.139)

I share her position that there is nothing more practical than to discover the patterns of movement and change that life requires. She cautions that our goal ought not be to crack the code of life (another existential issue), but rather advocates seeking to be able to sense the rhythm of life as change and ride with it. She asks how can descriptions that isolate, fragment, and objectify reality into parts of a system be considered practical compared to a continual improvement in understanding life as being so many relational, moving, learning variables be considered abstract (Bateson 2017)? Don't we create abstractions when we separate a person, idea, or organism from their many contextual relationships such as family, food, culture, feelings, ecology, and so on and label them? As with my concern regarding orthopedic complexity, it seems to me more abstract to take a piece of the living world and try to make sense of it without all the contexts that sustain health and function. Because of my shared frustration with Nora (I don't know Ms. Bateson, but I'm also quoting two other Batesons, hence the first name), we are shortly headed for a fascinating exploration around these *deep insights*, but first an appreciation for the role of paradox in wisdom.

Paradoxes

Paradoxes are a hallmark of integral and complex thinking. When you sense the discomfort of one, know you are probably on the right path rather the wrong path. We have dealt with a number so far in this book and there are many more ahead. I just want to spotlight them for a moment in case you begin to get paradox fatigue (not a real condition I can find anywhere). A paradox is two statements that appear to be a contradiction, but when examined from another perspective are not a contradiction after all. What? Our cultural habit of mind is dichotomous: this or that, it's either this or that, but not both. Our Western dualistic minds do not process paradoxes very well. Without a contemplative practice, our ability to hold creative tensions is very limited. Hence the common tendency to rush to judgment and demand a complete resolution of the tension with a polarized answer. The joke in my integral doctoral studies was that the right answer in any exam is always "both/and." It is both that and that. In order to fully understand paradoxes, we need to return to this idea of wisdom being developmental. If you haven't developed that far, the paradox will be an unsolvable riddle and, once you have developed wisdom, it will make complete sense at that new stage.

That means paradoxical understanding isn't a moral achievement or superior intellect, it is just the natural unfoldment of wisdom emerging over time. Rohr (2011) states that you and I are living paradoxes, and therefore must prepared to see ourselves in that reality. We are kind, yet impatient. We are wise and foolish. And on and on. He advises that if we can hold and forgive the contradictions within ourselves as a practice in paradoxes we can normally do it everywhere else. However, he cautions, if we cannot do it within ourselves, we will probably "create, project, and revel in dichotomies everywhere else in our lives" (2011, p.371).

Looks like we are back to our wisdom definition of *oneself*. We start with our self in dealing with paradox. In order to unlock a paradox, it always requires a change on the side of the observer, or us in this case. To arrive at an understanding of a paradox is to look at something long enough to get beyond the contradiction and see things at a different level of consciousness (transconceptually). This is often a primary and totally predictable effect of a transcendental yoga experience. The integrative effect of practice increases our awareness of not just us, but, because we're part of the bigger system of humankind, even the evolution of humanity, when we achieve a much higher capacity. Just as Sri Aurobindo (1993) suggests is our arc of evolution as both individuals and as a species.

As our development progresses, so too does our non-dual thinking. The dualistic dichotomies fall away so we also begin to see what we missed before. We no longer eliminate the negative, the problematic, or the threatening parts of everything. We don't divide the field of the present now, but receive it all. Our development allows a degree of real detachment from the small self, knowing that if what is present is true, it is its own best argument. This lack of the old polarized thinking trains us to hold creative tensions, which is to live with paradox and contradictions. Such tolerance reinforces how we shouldn't run from mystery and begin to be able to practice prosocial behaviors such as compassion, mercy, loving kindness, patience, forgiveness, and humility. Hang in there with all of these paradoxes. Embrace and accept what discomfort they may create knowing it is a very good step along our path of wisdom.

It is only fitting we conclude our brief discussion of paradoxes by considering another one: Everything new is old. Yes, things can be both old and new, and new and old.

Updating with Modern Wisdom and Yoga

I appreciate you sticking through this long chapter that at times might seem quite distant from learning some yoga for people in pain. I believe this next section is a linchpin in our transforming yoga therapy from an obscure, one of many, complementary care systems into a robust, easy to adopt care system for anyone. Without this chapter the wagon of yoga therapy might careen off into obscurity with no linchpin bringing its evolution along the course of time. It is that important. I am betting you will have a similar appreciation after you've completed this chapter.

The paradox of each being a part and a whole arises because our habitual way of understanding parts and wholes are ideas deeply imbedded beneath our conscious perception. Our entire industrial era way of knowing has been built on those notions, to include how we approach yoga. We therefore need to shine a spotlight onto the assumptions and many ways we communicate about our world. It is time to move beyond just Sanskrit and esoteric language and become conversant with modern culture. Note I didn't say eliminate Sanskrit. If we are going to be culturally competent and meet the needs of our populace we need to walk them here to our understanding versus try to get them to walk across a cultural chasm of language and culturally unfamiliar concepts and images.

Modern yoga and wisdom is emerging everywhere, but in modern language and inquiry. That's the entire point of the "old and new" paradox above. We have touched on this, but this chapter is where we learn our modern language of wisdom and yoga so that we can sew together (sutra?) our current culture and our beloved yoga tradition.

This is my best effort to find language that does exist, share the way it is used, and suggest how we as yoga professionals can/must adopt new words to communicate these important wisdom principles. The good news is there are such words. This won't be an exhaustive treatment, of course, but I hope it will prime you to continue to build and expand your vocabulary and that of those you serve. The process is both fun and inspiring. I will draw from just a few key resources based on their readability and modern orientation. In addition to Gregory and Nora Bateson, anthropologist Mary Catherine Bateson, Fr. Rohr (St. Francis taught integral theory), an Austrian-born, American physicist, Fritoj Capra, a psychiatrist, Daniel Siegel, and me. "Together" we'll cook up some new ways of understanding and saying our yoga teachings.

Please note, my motivation is not to completely bridge this enormous gap in cultures, but to simply deepen our understanding of both. I am not suggesting we will arrive at a final truth, but hopefully we will become more familiar with the many complexities that surround all that we study. We will never understand it completely or teach it completely, but we can create a lifelong habit of continually increasing our comprehension of the variables at play in successively pursuing *deep and accurate* insights.

Just as with my comments about Sanskrit, we aren't throwing out our dominant dualistic thinking either. In fact, non-dualistic thinking presumes that one has first mastered dualistic clarity, but found it insufficient for the central existential issues like love, suffering, death, God, and any notion of infinity. We need *both* kinds of thinking, that ongoing both/and integral refrain. We come to understand our world through knowledge, which is how we organize information. That's how we make sense of life, but our modern era is laboring under incomplete models of organization. That's why we see so much misunderstanding despite having a great deal of information freely available, with even more being created as big data.

Unfortunately, the dualistic current model of organizing the data lacks an ability to address the interrelationality between the data. Missing that yoga-ing thing. How do we describe information about relationships rather than just numbers? How do we describe how reality is woven together? How do we start to think accurately in a way that reflects that weave? (Hint: Context is key. The "text" is as in fabric or textile, the "con" is joining together.) That's what we get to create because that is what we're trying to sell as yoga professionals. No language, no communication: No sale.

A Simpler Way than Systems or Paradigm Shifts

I promised in the first yoga chapter not to overdo the *paradigm* word. I think the change we need to make isn't just our language and our actions, but also the logic or thinking formulation in which are actions are determined. Nora Bateson (2017) notes that, in our era of global crisis, too often there's talk of "paradigm shift" and "systems change" as being necessary for our biosphere and we as humans to survive. She argues there is another possibility, "The ingredient that I would like to add to the pot is the notion of life as mutual learning contexts" (p.166). We are going to explore that notion shortly. What if mutual learning takes place between all the parts, all the time in every situation or context? She advocates that asking from that notion recontextualizes all that has come before us and resets the horizon for understanding what will come in the future. I am excited about how this change in observing can take place, and, as a result, the way in which we can all begin to make observations through much more yogic lens. I am getting ahead of myself, but I wanted to assure you no complicated paradigm paragraphs lie ahead.

Panca Maya Kosha and BioPsychoSocialSpiritual as "Systems"

Our current use of systems such as the kosha model in yoga or the BPSS model in conventional healthcare will benefit from heeding Nora's argument. Our present habits of mind when trying to describe functioning parts and wholes is misleading and inaccurate for comprehending living, co-evolving systems. Metabolism, immunity, cognition, culture, and ecology are all examples of living interactions, as are suffering and pain. Our current teaching and description of these interactions fails to note the many perceptions, communications, and learning taking place in and between a complex tangle of varying perspectives.

For now, try to set aside your present understanding of your yoga and health models. Let's build a new vocabulary to begin to decrease the *superficialities and inaccuracies* in our study of living "systems" because they are very different from the mechanical ones most of our models are based upon. We will define systems related terminology and describe the benefits of adopting them, then clean up these errors about living systems in the "Cautions" section.

Definition of Systems

As we dive into systems and how they relate to yoga, it is good to remember that "being all one" is not the same as "being all the same." We yoga professionals are the integration specialists, and as such we aren't claiming everything is the same. Our role is to be able do more than just identify linkages that make us "one," but to also discern differences between. We want to move beyond a sense of separated, isolated different selves, but also honor our common ground (both/and). Optimal systems descriptions should allow us to sense our connections, our commonalities, as well as our differences. A system that can hold all three in fairly accurate representation will portray integration. More accurate systems maps can also go deep, pointing toward not only us connected to other people, but how we are connected to our common home, the Earth.

What makes for optimal systems descriptions? Ideally they would do what Gregory Bateson (2000) famously stated, and that is to be able to identify "the difference that makes a difference." The core of systems work isn't just accumulated details of data, but patterns of relationship. This is not easy for our Western culture as I have mentioned several times. Our habit of applying ideas of cause and effect for the past 400-plus years to cultural, scientific, and theological development has been responsible for many positive developments. Good systems thinking allows us to see past those old formulas and begin to peer into the world of interrelations versus straight line causality. There don't appear to be quite as many straight lines of cause and effect after all. Systems thinking will require us to discontinue that well-ingrained habit and learn to be willing to look in many directions at once and then articulate numerous (countless?) patterns of interaction. As yogic systems thinkers, we will alter our perspectives beyond just quantity of data, to quality of "how" data is related. The themes will be changing from objects to relationships, from just measuring to mapping in refined and varied detail, and from just more quantity to quality of ever growing quantity.

As you can see this change is not the easy route. No glib declarations or trite witticisms. Gone are the quick solutions. The complexity thought process demands a more engaged exploration of the patterns that connect. Bottom line, quick short cuts miss critical relationships, generating *superficial and inaccurate answers,* and ultimately lead to *unskillful, less than benevolent responses.* Does this explanation weave you back into the wisdom definition and how it applies to our best modern complexity thinking? I think it is fascinating and worth wading into deeply.

A bonus to this wading is that our deeper understanding of how the incredible range of variables and interactions in the natural world are functioning then also informs our actions or *responsiveness.* You and your students will then be better informed around the ethics within the yamas and niyamas, the subsequent choices of skilled actions, and a deeper awareness for why we make those choices. Were we to just superficially declare we are all the same and one based on a superficial unity model, we would lose what Bateson (2017, p.97) describes as "the differences, the information, the aesthetics of interaction, the evolution, the complexity," and the dynamism of life. So remember, Unity with the capital "U" is not about oneness. Unity requires a process both of uniting despite differences and of linking through understanding relationality. How do we construct optimal systems of relationships that communicate the critical contrasts within unity? I am glad you asked.

Transcontextuality

First we had transconceptual, now transcontextual arrives to assist our complex thinking and sensing skills. Ordinarily subjects under study or description don't get to bring along their relationships, and the contexts get lost in the data. I can remember something as simple as writing a report on a hammerhead shark. I had so much data on the size, weight, diet, and location of the shark. I even remember drawing the picture for the cover, a form in isolation on a bed of blue. Where'd the context go? Why did it live where it did? Why were its eyes out like that? I know I wrote where they were positioned, but no context for why. How was it related to the other sharks? Why didn't it exist elsewhere? In hindsight, I can see that just the context I shared was not enough. Bateson (2017, p.160) states that, "living systems especially require more than one context of study if we're to get a grasp of their vitality."

Transcontextual description is when we examine the interdependency that characterizes living systems. The "trans" (over and through) multiple lens of context create a transcontextual lens. Where one context interfaces with others is where that mutual learning I mentioned earlier takes place. Such a lens offers entirely new dimensions of information that can help us know so much more about situation than any single plane or a single context would reveal. Regarding the shark's food source: What was the evolutionary circumstance that made the shape of the hammerhead advantageous evolutionarily? Was that advantage still present or was species adaptation or depletion putting the shark at risk? Were there new food sources where the shark had migrated because of warming waters? Did that migration offer nutritional gains or shortcomings? Was the shark having to learn new feeding strategies and was that a stress that affected reproduction?

Can you sense all the different dimensions compared to my flat single plane shark with some data? Notice how as I dug deeper through multiple descriptive processes I gained sight of the many new perspectives that required integrating. Transcontextuality is extremely rigorous when done well. And, to be done well, it requires more than just my perspectives.

Imagine what a colleague with marine science expertise could add, or a climate change specialist? When we get to the pain and creativity chapters, these multiple inputs are key and hint at the value of sangha/community in wisdom development and systems understanding. The both/and of the individual and the whole of the community. Because life is transcontextual by definition, only transcontextual observation offers the most basic practical understanding of nature, which as in wisdom, starts with our own existence as individuals.

Transcontextual observation blurs the sharp outlines of parts, as the identifiable "roles" of the parts and wholes within the function of a system are revealed to be contextual. The part description of that hammerhead's head and eyes now seems so flat and lifeless. Can you sense how your identity is also not singular in context? You may be friends to some people, classmates to others, parents to your children and the child of your parents, and co-workers at your job. Despite all those contexts, aren't you also just still yourself? Isn't it fun how once we start to use that transcontextual lens, the world unfolds in so many new dimensions? Between each of your roles at those interfaces, isn't there also new learning that you acquired while at the same time the others in that interface were having to mutually learn from relating with you?

Sadly, when we habitually remove ambiguity from situations, we also simultaneously remove transcontextual information. The day the marine biologists tracked the shark's consumption it ate a certain kind of fish. Therefore, hammerheads eat those fish. But wait, are those fish always present? What did it eat yesterday and last summer? That's too ambiguous, we need to cut this diet description off right: Here. Ironically, Bateson (2017) says ambiguity provides more insight to us via additional transcontextual information that allows for more ways to appreciate and nuance more graceful actions as a result. Limited ambiguity, limited potentially stilted choices miss valuable relationships. This leaves us with another paradox that more blurry description is actually clearer and vice versa. Certainly the loss of sharp outlines and certainty is uncomfortable, but, as we keep discovering, that certainty was an illusion all along.

When we talk about pain soon, there will be so many blurry descriptions beyond anatomical parts and visible tissue changes. Just to consider general cultural and familial tendencies around pain and suffering, let alone specifics to a student will be almost impossible to pin down. The "I" you sit across from in teaching lives in a body that internally requires co-existence with more than 10 trillion organisms, as do you, while both of you are immersed in your own survival within a complex ecology, imbued with emotion and shifting societal values. Do you see how flat and lifeless teaching that sacral adjustment block trick is now for the person with chronic back pain? You are going to love all the benefits this complex systems thinking will offer you. Sure, it is harder work, but wisdom would be much more prevalent if it was easy, wouldn't it?

Benefits of Systems and Complexity Thinking

The hard work of this type of thinking unearths the very structures upon which we build our ideas. Just seeing that complexity allows one to give up the concrete certainty and be open to new perspectives. My thinking about my thinking (metacognition) also reveals my motivations, giving me an opportunity to monitor the *benevolence* factor of my actions. The complexity of my discoveries won't necessarily help me solve a specific problem, but it should decrease the risk for harm despite my best intentions. A real joy is when we discover the deep ideas that have become invisible to us because of how they're integrated into our lives. Without such a discovery, our ideas can feel unchangeable, but, as Bateson kindly offers, "But, pull a single thread loose and the whole tapestry can be reorganized" (2017, p.22). Thus many new possibilities open up in what felt immutable, making the effort worthwhile.

Another benefit is how this thinking assists us in addressing the *oneself* of the *deep and accurate insights* of wisdom. Again, Bateson (2017) points out that just the grammar of asking "Who am I?" inaccurately suggests that the "I" in question is singular. Consider the complexity when she rightly points out that the complexity of a human is lost because there is no plural first person that we know must be there given everything we have been discussing in this chapter. "That singularity is a semantic, ideological, epistemological, cultural, biological, ecological, evolutionary, epigenetic, gender specific, nationalistic error" (2017, p.25). Can you feel the flatness of you as I, compared to the multiplane dimensions of what is lost without complexity thinking? No wonder we struggle with the *oneself* half of the wisdom definition when we are searching for the asmitâ-like "I" as an independent individual instead of the complex, interdependent shifting being that reflects reality. Feel both the relief of discovery, but also the weight of responsibility for us and those we serve.

Once we begin to see the complexities of "I," we also start to glimpse and can't help noticing the complexities of others. These create many surprises as relationships and new meanings generate both small and big shifts of meaning and understanding. As members of a student's web of care providers, ideally we then begin to see and appreciate new aspects of the team and how it can support the student. This is the goal of interprofessional dialogue that is a nice concept but often fails to take place because of our imbedded and unexamined ideas about other professions. That of course is a form of violence then toward the one we are trying to serve. What would happen if we all adopted this complex form of inquiry and communication as a value system of "courageous affection" (Bateson 2017, p.45) for other professions rather than the societal competitor perspective that dominates? I can't see who would lose in such a community, can you?

We live in a time where the English language is nearly devoid of words that communicate what we yoga professionals are trying to sell: integral (all part of one) understanding. This bears repeating. All this wisdom and yoga stuff, and we don't have common words to describe or communicate the principles effectively. That's a problem. Nora Bateson (2017) uses the word "ecologies" as a way to point to multiplicity within the realities we live. She writes of the ecology of the individual, the family, the culture, of relating humans, and of our interaction with what we call nature. The more care and attention we give to our language choices, the more powerfully we can relate to loosen the knot of tangles, and, for this book, the knot of pain and suffering.

How you language what you are discovering by reading this book will determine the quality of relationships you establish in your future teaching. We are all language dependent. Let's seize the power of *skillful* language choices.

With Power There Are Cautions

The problem with this darn complexity and systems thinking is we then have to know there are potential perils to using it. Ambiguity everywhere. The invisible ideas we have beneath what systems are can impede or completely corrupt our use of systems. Our societal bias with systems is that of assembling all the parts of what we are contemplating, then arranging them in orders until every part is diagrammed within some "whole" that we believe we are applying systems thinking to. Unfortunately, that is a mechanistic, linear (even if the arrows point in several directions) explanation via a reductionistic diagram. We can't offer multiplanar insights around the mutual learning and co-evolution that takes place simultaneously in living systems with a flat, two-dimensional depiction without losing the messiness and transcontextual relationships. More violence. The psycho changes the bio of BPS, or the ananda influences the prana of the koshas, but how do we depict the immediate reverse influence those "parts" have not only on one another, or the other components of the system in consideration, but what of the changes and learning in the larger system in which that individual is imbedded? Again, our models become flat, dry, and lifeless, but they are tidy to gaze upon. The loss of complexity and messiness also leads to more *superficial and inaccurate insights*, steering us away from wisdom and *skillful responses*. Bateson (2017) correctly points out what is lost are the many layers of learning that are always taking place, whether it's a family, jungle, or business organization. Just making correlations between some parts be they BPSSs or koshas isn't enough, we need more skills.

How then can we see the interactions and interrelationships more skillfully? You guessed it, we're back at another paradox. When we label parts with "their" functions, we also assign agency or power as though it arises out of the specific part. Once we do that, we begin to lose accuracy as the parts bleed away the actual power of the ecology of larger systems. Bateson writes, "Agency implies that parts can be separated from wholes and exert individuated action" (2017, p.174). She suggests that agency ought to be treated as a paradox that exists between the statement that the existence of the organism is a unique entity *and* the "simultaneous impossibility that this entity can be decontextualized or in any way uninfluenced by its contextual interactions" (p.174). Can you see how the concept of agency for an entity blurs within this paradox of what seems to be two true statements that contradict one another? While this may be uncomfortable and raise doubts about how an individual can ever then relieve their suffering and pain, it also suggests bold new possibilities for how we learn together. For now, just be careful not to mix up the uniqueness of each of us with a single purpose or agency of that unique entity imagined as independence. Asmitâ again. She hopes we can just allow this paradox to co-exist and resist the temptation to solve it.

What then are we to do with these limitations of systems and complexity thinking? Because the English language lacks the words to describe such thinking, I believe learning a short list of related terms will increase our understanding substantially and enable us to communicate more effectively within our respective communities. Think of this as learning the Sanskrit names for asana. Not terribly fun, but how it deepened your understanding of the asana to be able to communicate more accurately within the yoga community.

Words to Know

Symmathesy

First a big one with a longer explanation. The remainder are much more succinct, but this word of Nora Bateson's (2017) creation in my opinion is very important. We seek to avoid the dangerous habit of describing complex systems in terms of parts and wholes. We have described the loss of mutual learning in engineering diagrams. How then do we describe the multiple levels of learning within context? That's the word we need to communicate a new systemic vision, a vision that sees life as relational, mutual learning contexts. Disciplines from pain science, epigenetics, social science, economic theory, and evolutionary theory all demonstrate that evolution emerges in relationships, not in a linear fashion. Gregory Bateson (2000) wrote that we discover the evolution in the context. The need for a word that describes the constant learning and communication in living systems resulted in Nora combining two Greek words, *syn/sym* (together) and *mathesi* (to learn), to create symmathesy (learning together) (Bateson 2017, p.169). Consider, as I describe this word, does it fill in a gap in this communication puzzle we've been exploring? It does for me.

As a noun, she offers that it is an entity that forms over time by contextual mutual learning through interaction. Symmathesy is the *process*. Hmmm, where did we see this definition before, perhaps in defining yoga therapy? As a verb, she modifies it to symmathesize, which is when the process takes place between multiple variables in a living entity. Because this word describes the interlearning within the whole, to move away from the mechanistic parts of engineering, she offers one other word for the living parts: *vita* (plural: *vitae*): She defines vita as "any aspect of a living entity that, through interfaces of learning, forms a larger living entity or symmathesy. For example, the 'members' of a family, organs in the body, or flora and fauna in a forest" (p.169).

That's it for made up words. But can you appreciate how they fill in an important communication gap? For me it provides a lens where I begin to look for and see interrelational context, communication, and learning. This symmathesy also provides a sense of the glue-of-relationship that holds the system together through time and into its evolution. This can be the symmathesy of a synapse in the nervous system, the symmathesy of a poisoned family dynamic, or the symmathesy of an executive committee of a multinational corporation polluting the environment. The neuropeptides, synaptic membrane and space, the family members and ancestors, and the consumers, shareholder, and board of directors are all aspects of those living entities. Each learning, adapting, and evolving in and from a myriad of directions. This new ability to increase the depth and richness of a more precise way of thinking is tremendously exciting for me. There is power in our words, and if chosen well we can go deeper and more accurately in our pursuit of wisdom. Symmathesy is just such a term, that brings clarity and complexity to our thoughts about life and its *existential issues*, putting them into the fabric (text) of relation to each other, and in those relationships there is a state of constant learning and change.

Learning

Not a new word, but one that deserves updating, just like the software on your phone, as use changes over time. Typically learning is used to denote acquiring knowledge across time both intellectually and physically. With the advent of using symmathesy, learning will include the entire living world as a context of learning since we now appreciate that mutual learning doesn't stop at the skin of the entity, nor does it only involve the intellectual and physical performance of the entity. The world is now understood to be a "symmathesy composed of symmathesies" (Bateson 2017). This learning isn't necessarily "good" or "bad" as it includes both adaptation, maladaptation, and even addiction. The kaleidoscope of so many shifting calibrations, adjustments, new patterns makes learning closer to co-evolution, provided we don't take the learning to necessarily mean "progress" or improvement. As we will see shortly in Chapter 4, we can be very good at learning to generate pain too.

Consider some of the characteristics of learning in symmathesy and the new use for old words we can employ (Bateson 2017):

Contexts: The internal and external interactions that create contexts within which the entity exists. Remember, think: Con (together) + text (fabric, textile).

Calibration: The precise and continuous adjustments within contexts of many interrelated variables. Calibrations aren't necessarily conscious and can be the "difference that makes a difference."

Bias: The bias in the calibrations of the entity at every scale. These biases affect the particular integration of the many variables of interrelating information influencing our focus, the person. The bias forms differences. The individual has multiple interfaces, and a bias through that filters and frames, on an ongoing basis, the information they are calibrating. They can be structural, not just conceptual in pain and suffering.

Stochastic: (Unpredictable) process is randomly determined, but may not be predicted precisely. This relates to the emergence and surprise of complex living systems. The entity may appear stable, but random inputs and the implicit variables between the many vitae of a symmathesy are ultimately unpredictable. There is both pattern and unpredictability. Watching our own and our students' behavior should offer many example of the stochastic nature of symmathesies. Watch the Minnesota Adventure unfold as an example.

Play: Play is our way of learning to learn. It can be in the forms of games, humor, art, experimenting, fighting, attempting, reorganizing, and yoga technologies. Practice, repetition, and experimentation in communication and behavior around the edges of a bias are the frontiers of such learning, evolution, and change. It is also where yoga practice interfaces with suffering. Hence you keep seeing me use the word "fun."

Boundaries: Boundaries are the interfaces of learning around the edge of the context. They are not static and in themselves represent another paradox of "an edge but not an edge" because of the constant change as time flows while the various contexts continue to interact and learn. Where is the edge of comfortable movement limitation? And how about now? And now? Slippery boundaries.

Time: Can be described as the phenomenon that arises with the observed flow of change and learning. All living organisms and vitae exist within a context of mutual learning, revealing that order is not static across "time." Another definition of "suffer" is to allow across time. Pain changes across time and isn't static. So many fun aspects to learn.

Life: The emerging new scientific conception of life is seen as part of a broader world view shift from a mechanistic to a holistic and ecological worldview (Capra and Luisi 2016). Nuanced by the classic view of life, in fact the root meaning of both the Greek *psyche* and the Latin *anima* is "breath." Closely associated with that moving force, the breath of life that leaves the body at death, was the idea of knowing and learning. For the early Greek philosophers, the soul was both the source of movement and life, and that which perceives and knows through continual learning. Also defined as life = change; from a systems view, a structurally coupled system is a learning system. Life is continual structural changes in response to the environmental changes and requiring continuing adaptation, learning, and development as key characteristics of the behavior of all living entities: Pointing us toward context. Does this remind anyone of prana and other yoga terminology around kundalini, oja, and so on?

Entropy versus health/life: Biological evolution means a movement toward increasing order and complexity; in physics it came to mean just the opposite – a movement toward increasing disorder/entropy (Capra and Luisi 2016). That was classical thermodynamics with its celebrated "second law" of the dissipation of energy. The living world is now understood to be an unfolding toward increasing order and complexity and not that of running down into ever-increasing disorder.

Ecology: The totality or pattern of relations between organisms and their environment (Capra and Luisi 2016). Ecology is the totality of patterns of interrelationship that form interdependencies. Not just that chapter in biology about life at the pond or being green in our environmental practices.

Eco-literacy = health? The new appreciation that larger systems are not ordered above the smaller ones in pyramid fashion (Capra and Luisi 2016). Rather, in nature, there is no "above" or "below," and there are no hierarchies. Just networks nesting within other networks. This systems view of life is an ecological view that is grounded, ultimately, in spiritual awareness (Who am I?, What am I?, and How shall I act or be?). The fundamental concepts of ecology are connectedness, relationship, and community. Those three concepts are the essence of spiritual experience. Maybe yoga professionals are eco-literacy teachers as well as purveyors of a psychospiritual science? Think about it.

Emergence: The essential properties of a living system are emergent properties (Capra and Luisi 2016). By emergent I mean properties that are not found in any of the parts but emerge at the level of the system as a whole. They arise from specific patterns of organization expressed in configurations of ordered relationships among the vitae. Rather than rigid, these systems are said to be structurally unstable, and the critical points of instability are called "bifurcation points." These are the points in the system's evolution where a fork suddenly appears and the system branches off in a new direction. Physically, the bifurcation points correspond to points of instability at which the system changes abruptly and new forms of order suddenly appear (surprise, not predicted). This spontaneous emergence of order at critical points of instability is a hallmark of life. In non-linear dynamics (i.e., living systems) simple equations may generate enormously complex strange attractors, and simple rules of iteration give rise to structures more complicated than we can even imagine. Emergence, in the most classic interpretation, means in fact the arising of novel properties in an ensemble, novel in the sense that they are not present in the constituents. As scientists peer into how life might have started they arrive at yet another paradox. On the one hand, they say that biological life is chemistry only; on the other hand, they also state that the arising of life as a property cannot be reduced to the properties of the single chemical components present. More ambiguity as far back as we can see.

Relationships science: I love Capra and Luisi's *A Systems View of Life* (2016). These are some more pearls from their exhaustive work. Living systems cannot be understood by analysis alone. The properties of the vitae are not intrinsic properties, but can be understood only within the context of the larger whole. That means the relationship between the parts and the whole has been reversed. A systems approach acknowledges the properties of the parts can be understood only from the organization of the whole. This shifts the systems thinking to not focus on basic building blocks but rather on basic principles of organization: Another way of saying systems thinking is "contextual," the opposite of analytical thinking. Analysis means taking something apart in order to understand it; systems thinking means putting it into the context of a larger whole. They ask, "What does the term 'systems view' mean when it is applied to life?", to which they answer that it implies looking at a living organism in the totality of its mutual interactions. You've heard this several times, but it is so important in the remainder of the book.

Uncertainty: What makes it possible to turn the systems approach into a proper science is the discovery that there is approximate knowledge (Capra and Luisi 2016). This *insight* is crucial to all contemporary science. In the systemic worldview it is recognized that all scientific concepts and theories (theater?) are limited and approximate. Science can never provide any complete and definitive understanding. Going back to breaking down the yoga definitions, I tried to convey that we never deal with truth, in the sense of a precise correspondence between our descriptions and the described phenomena. We always deal with limited and approximate knowledge. And so do our students and the community we serve.

Feedback: Feedback has come to mean the delivery of information about the outcome of any process or activity to its source (Capra and Luisi 2016). What if there is no single source and the entire system is mutually learning? That is a non-linear, complex system, where, by contrast, small changes may have dramatic effects because they may be amplified repeatedly by self-reinforcing feedback. Such non-linear feedback processes are the basis of the instabilities and the sudden emergence of new forms of order that are so characteristic of self-organization and emergence. When we train others to focus and attend to internal feedback, that attention can prime the system for the creativity of emergence.

Autopoiesis: *Auto*, of course, means "self" and refers to the autonomy of self-organizing systems, and *poiesis* (which shares the same Greek root as the word "poetry") means "making" (Capra and Luisi 2016). So autopoiesis means "self-making." This is the main characteristic of life and occurs as self-maintenance due to the internal networking of a living chemical system that continuously reproduces itself within a boundary of its own making. This self-maintenance is via a mechanism of self-regeneration from within. It can be said that life is a factory that makes itself from within. That's good news because that includes making pain and suffering, only in modern scientific language.

So what? Not a new use of words, but the question you might well ask after digging so deeply into this topic. Bateson (2017) used the example of a hand several times to offer a so what. I will as well, but from our context as readers of this book. Vitae such as your dominant hand interface in multiple contexts. Your ability to observe your own hand and hold simultaneous contextual descriptions of the hand will provide you a deeper and more complex understanding of "hand." We make this understanding more valuable if the contexts or sets of relationships of that vita are brought into the description. Within the form you refer to as your hand, what communicative and information processes bring together the many contextual ecologies and provide the fodder for symmathesy? Gazing upon my dominant left hand there many levels. The swollen index knuckle from high school basketball, the sliver of wood imbedded still from climbing Mr. Wilsey's fence, the scars from the razor from trimming my model planes in junior high are just a few artifacts of interfaces my hand was a part of. The callus at the base of my wedding band points to a 40-year relationship with my wife. The absence of other calluses to the fact that I earned my living thinking rather than with hard manual labor. The gray hairs amongst the black speak to 59 years of living.

If I was able to scan my brain on the right side I'd find different movement and sensing maps by structure and function than what supply my right hand on the left side of my brain. The interface with a pen or fork is superior on the left, but the interfaces are inferior on the right regarding computer mice and scissors. That inferiority is cultural due to right-handed bias for both of those tools, but define my "hand." My left hand knows my left ear much better than the right by its position on my body and tendency to use same side hands to scratch or wash each ear. My left hand is able to generate more force pounds than the right. My hand doesn't start at my wrist, as many nerves, arteries and veins, tendons and ligaments extend up my forearm. My ability to perceive with my hand doesn't stop at my skin and also goes deep within my bones. My hand doesn't move of its own accord, but complies (usually) with my intentions and motor messages. Sometimes it feels big and sometimes small, even though by sight it appears unchanged. The genetics that drove the formation of my hand extend in an unbroken chain of evolutionary development for over one million years. Your turn now. Describe the countless interfaces of learning and change that make up what you used to define as your dominant hand. Have fun.

And the Qualities to Have

There will be many exercises to stimulate your ability to see more complexly in the practice chapter. I hope the hand exercise gave you a good glimpse into the wealth of relationships available that were probably overlooked by a parts dominance in the past. There are a few qualities for you to carry forward that will also supplement your complexity practices. First, there is humility. We mentioned three forms of humility earlier this chapter when we discussed accuracy as a part of wisdom. Revisit those if you don't recall. The present-day arrogance of scientific philosophy is now proving obsolete, and in its place, there is the discovery we are describing here that humans are only a part of larger systems and that the part can never control the whole. As we address large systems challenges, we will be well served to remember that.

Related to humility, be careful not to presume any of us can plot trajectory, let alone predict a future that can be controlled. We will do better to remain sensitive to the aesthetic, making small shifts in the ecology across multiple layers at the level of context. This won't be easy, as we mentioned about wisdom in general. It will require a rigor of intellect, perception, and emotional flexibility and sensitivity. This isn't about romantically just letting things happen. No, we need to develop the rigor necessary to hold variables in focus despite the blurry unknown. Bateson cautions, "To take into account the larger consequences of our 'actions' is to better understand the many facets of our interactions" (2017, p.189).

We also touched on organizational yoga therapy last chapter. Using our new constructs and terms, is it easy to see our institutions function very much like a forest or an ocean in their life and complexity? The infrastructures of our institutions reinforce and balance one another, and our socioeconomic system develops in patterns that fit the characteristics of any ecology. Consider how technology, shopping, and entertainment are woven together at so many levels now. When we participate, we are contributing perfectly to that very ecology that we live within. How might these ideas of contextual organizational rehabilitation help us to address the dysfunctional and fixed interrelationships within the ecology of institutions? Wouldn't it be nice if we could address the context of these institutions instead of attempting to chase down crisis after crisis as separate issues (Bateson 2017)? We fool ourselves if we believe we can limit our yoga profession to working with just individuals. And, as I hinted, the way to shift systems is through guiding creative practice by those very same individuals that make up the systems. Us.

Another point highlighting the asmitâ-itis I mentioned much earlier. Did you know botanists don't describe the ecology and evolution of individual plants, but of "holobionts," entities made of many species, all inseparably linked (Haskell 2017)? Biologists now know that living networks are ancient, perhaps as old as life itself. Models and lab experiments on the chemical origin of life show that interacting, "cooperating" networks of molecules beat self-replicating molecules in a Darwinian struggle. So just as our pain isn't ours alone, neither is our healing as an inseparably linked network. The fundamental unit of biology is not the "self," but the network. A pine tree is actually a plurality, its "individuality" a temporary composition of relationships. Life can be described as a busy conversation, embodied, in a mutual learning network. To put it succinctly, any sense of self we have is really a society (Haskell 2017). The rediscovery of the misdirection of asmitâ.

It bears repeating that Gregory Bateson, renowned anthropologist and polymath (knew a great deal across a wide range of disciplines), points us in a good focus with "The difference that makes a difference." Those simple words described his lifetime of foraging for language changes to comprehend and communicate wisdom. He sought to have others explore with him the nuances and small differences that had big effects on the many systems that woven together. If you can mine a word or expression that allows a student to "see" or experience a new relationship of connection with their suffering, that's a difference that makes a difference. For instance, guiding them to experience how their breath changes and throat tightens when someone speaks over them at work might be the difference that leads not only to fewer late day headaches, but emboldens them to speak up, seek new communication skills, or leave that environment. That early warning embodied experience could be the small difference that makes all the difference. But if you can't communicate effectively, the opportunity will be lost.

What is it we're trying to communicate? Bateson's daughter, Nora, another polymath in her own right, has both the science and the art of describing what often feels like the indescribable we are seeking. Pause, then read her quote below and sense what you experience through the power of ordinary words to describe the ordinary, very yoga concept she describes:

> In the kitchen, in the street, in the forest, in the sea, in my cells and in the cache of breaths I cannot count—there is something holding all of this together, all of us together. There is an alive order that we are within and that is within us. (Bateson 2017, p.17)

What did you sense? Did it feel familiar? Was there a sense of arriving home? Other than "cache," all of the words were simple. In her book *Small Arcs of Larger Circles* (2017) she is building the kind of language we need. Some, as we saw, are new words, most, though, just new ways of saying wise principles with common words. That's a quality we should all seek to express. Let's start by considering some implications that this deep study of wisdom, old and new, has primed us to adopt in our yoga profession.

Yoga Implications

Last chapter we discussed word choices and reading across different disciplines in order to be more effective in saying it to more people. As I researched the wisdom literature I discovered these yoga related pearls to help you build your collections.

Yoga definitions of wisdom: Even within our yoga, wisdom has been described through translation several ways. Patanjali Yoga Sutra 2.27 describes the final unceasing vision of discernment as wisdom (prajna). The next sutra, 2.28, then states that our goal through the performance of the limbs of Yoga, and with the dwindling of impurity is the radiance of wisdom (jnana), [which develops, or is a developmental model] up to the vision of discernment (Feuerstein 1998, p.297). Elsewhere wisdom (jnana) and action (karma) are compared to two wings of the same bird and noted that emancipation is achieved by the harmonious development of both means in order for the bird to fly (Feuerstein 1998, p.66). Finally, as another tiny sample, the Yoga-Vasishtha, composed a thousand years after the Bhagavad-Gita, declares, "Karma-Yoga is the most grounded of all yogic approaches" (Feuerstein 1998, p.67). Given these many definitions just from yoga I don't understand how Walsh wrote such a succinct but meaningful summary definition of wisdom.

Mind defined: Chitta, buddhi, manas, rita-cit, etc. Now we can celebrate that the decisive advance of the systems view of life has been to abandon the Cartesian (separate parts/mechanistic) view of mind as a thing, and to realize that mind and consciousness are not things but processes. Further, that mind is manifest not only in individual organisms but also in social systems and ecosystems (Capra and Luisi 2016). Never *mind* trying to find something new.

Could these be Indryas? Maturana and Varela, two twentieth-century "yogis" of systems theory experts, stated that the organism interacts with the environment in a "cognitive" (jnana) way whereby the organism "creates" (karma) its own environment and the environment simultaneously permits the actualization of the organism. From the hills of Kashmir to South America to your eyes. Something old is new again.

Pratyahara: Again, Maturana and Varela note that we can never direct a living system. They believe, because of the agency of the system, that it can only be disturbed. More than that, the living system not only specifies its structural changes, but it also specifies which disturbances from the environment trigger the structural changes. In other words, a living system has the autonomy to discriminate what to notice and what will disturb it. We are going to see a great deal of this in the pain chapter coming up next. I wonder what practice might help?

Seer and the seen: There's a constant tension between being part of the whole and an individual. The double role of living systems as parts and wholes requires the interplay of two opposite tendencies: An integrative tendency to function as part of a larger whole, and a self-assertive, or self-organizing tendency to preserve individual autonomy. Notice how the language describes in modern terminology this age-old paradox you almost certainly explored in your training and most likely teach to your students.

Panca maya kosha: This chapter has trumpeted our need to change to systems/koshas thinking, those koshas being so much bigger than within the skin and skull of the anna/food/physical body now. Systems thinking means a shift of perception from material objects and structures to the non-material processes and patterns of organization that represent the very essence of life. Exercises ahead.

Asmitâ in twentieth-century physics? Renowned physicist Werner Heisenberg (1958, p.58) stated, "What we observe is not nature itself, but nature exposed to our method of questioning." Therefore transconceptual wisdom offers an escape from the vrittis/misperceptions of the our mind that generate asmitâ. Too quickly we forget or become ignorant (avidyâ) that life is not localized within our lens. Life is a global property, arising from the collective interactions of reality and subject to deep contemplation and reflection. Always question our lens when considering self and reality. It's probably dirty.

Death: Hey, I'm married to a death educator. You didn't think you were going to get out this book without discussing death, did you? Death is *the* central existential issue (Taylor 2008). As they say, "Ain't none of us getting out of here alive" (author unknown). One death, at the level of our individual life, is aging. The other death, at the level of the progression of generations in time, is evolution. These are described as the two irreversible arrows of time, and each one has its own characteristic features. The end of aging is death, a process by which all molecular components are yielded back to the environment, and used for other purposes. Entire species are undergoing the sixth known great extinction as you read. Death breathes down our collective neck as the environment groans under human generated stress. (I'm guessing I lost all of the climate change deniers a couple chapters back.) Abhinivesha is a klesha because we avoid her. We do so at our literal peril and risk of future suffering.

Karma yoga: Wisdom reveals that we can inspire others by how we ourselves live our lives. A common statement in wisdom traditions, now affirmed by careful research in a range of scientific disciplines is that, if you want to be happy, help others. Reciprocally, if you want others to be happy, help others. When we integrate the chaos and rigidity in our lives through service to the other and it becomes a central drive, we cultivate meaning and connection, happiness and health (Siegel 2017). Being able to wisely differentiate oneself from others, and then link to them by serving to support their wellbeing, is a win–win. This balance not only of compassionate care, but also the empathic joy of the interpersonal experience of savoring others' successes in life which are Patanjali's sutras in action. Wisdom reveals that being human is a journey of discovery, a process that empowers us to embrace such yoking/integration as a principle. Skillful action (yoga) means we set an intention toward integration/yoking without being committed to some specific outcome or result. This intention invites new mutual learning (Bateson 2017), moment by moment. Our job ahead is to cultivate a deep sense of connection and satisfaction, and perhaps even meaning and purpose as we serve. Siegel (2017, p.209) admonishes that "Wisdom is something that can arise within each of us and be shared by us all."

Yoga memes and rockstars: Have you noticed what passes for wisdom in the popular yoga community? Presumably wisdom is not tweeting dubious Buddha quotes, pretty memes with pop psychology references, and the whole "yoga of abundance" trend. Our culture of consumerism makes it difficult to discern wisdom from stardom. It is our responsibility to discern with our new-found understanding of wisdom, first whether we are behaving wisely with *skillful, benevolent responsiveness* in our personal lives, and then as yoga professionals. This is important work and I think it will require constant reappraisal. As I type these words, I am checking again why I am spending this beautiful autumn morning indoors staring at this screen? Am I trying to be an authority or sage? Do I want public acclaim or notoriety? Apparently I've told myself some other story, because I am still typing. Just as in our yoga therapy definition, the discernment we exercise when we ask whether we are empowering ourselves and those we serve is an important wisdom practice. If I become someone else's authority, is that wise? If someone wants me to be their authority, is that wisdom? There's much work to be done in our yoga community around this fine discrimination. Are we offering a coherent message that empowers the individual? Wisdom seeing has always sought to change the seer first, and then knows that what is seen will largely take care of itself. To quote Fr. Rohr (2011, p.152), "It is almost that simple, and it is always that hard."

What other yoga themes did you discover in this chapter? Add them to your list. They're everywhere and so fun to collect.

Spiritual Implications

I mentioned in the first yoga chapter about my former nice, neat compartmentalized life. It included one compartment titled "Spiritual Life." The labeling suggests it was distinct and separate from the rest of my life. Many of us still maintain those divisions and I suspect many of those we teach do as well, if they even acknowledge having a spiritual life. One of my early breakthroughs of the walled sections came when Fr. Mike Librandi, a dear friend and my pastor at the time, introduced me to progressive theological writers. That introduction was hard on my certainty, but was a true spark of transforming my understanding and yielded so many insights throughout the former compartments. If you can glimpse some relationships between your spiritual practice, that of your students, and that of general audiences and how the practices can be described in terms of wisdom, I am hoping those descriptions will allow you to create bridges and gateways between the artificial separations that might be generating suffering now.

The foundational spiritual questions are part of the existential issues of life in our definition of wisdom. Those questions are, "Who am I?", "What am I?", and, based on those answers, "How shall I act or be in life?" When we invite students to participate in first-person ethical reviews and the studies of the yamas and niyamas, that's a spiritual inquiry. Regardless of whether they have a religious practice, those are wisdom questions that deal directly with establishing deep accurate insight of themselves. Their lived experience in light of those answers describes their current life work or dharma. If there's coherence and resonance, there's apt to be much less suffering. If there's little or no alignment, as described by Sullivan *et al.* (2017), such a review may be very powerful in identifying some of the sources of their suffering. This inquiry can be done secularly, devoid of religious connection or placed alongside their personal religious beliefs and practices. Incongruities and dissonance are understood to distress an overactive mind, dysregulate emotions, and adversely affect prosocial and skillful behaviors sought in the *skillful benevolent responsiveness* of wisdom. The spiritual practice lies in contemplation, reflection, reordering ethics, and then behaving in accordance with those changes. Simple in description, potentially very challenging in practice.

One of the big insights I gained in my process of reading the progressive teachers was the role of power and gender in modern day religion. Historical review finds that wisdom/sophia/chokmah and many other names for wisdom were generally feminine in nature and referred to as feminine. This contrasted sharply with the patriarchal and masculine religious practice that was my experience. Each person will have their own unique insight and discoveries in their inquiry, so we should be careful not to project or direct our views. Rather, by inviting and when appropriate, helping them procure appropriate spiritual direction if need be, the ground is prepared for the emergence of wisdom specific to their circumstance. Discovering the yoga energies of the polarities, whether masculine/feminine, light/dark, suffering/resurrection, and on and on, all four forms of wisdom are primed to be discovered and experienced. How practical, intuitive, conceptual or transconceptual wisdom shows up will often be a surprise and a delight. Uncertainty restricts from predicting, but rather invites surrendering to the mystery through the niyama of ishvara pranidhana in a way that matches them best. I cannot fathom any asana directly bringing that depth of transformation that is both transconceptual and transcendent.

Pain Crisis

What in the world does it mean to teach from the wisdom of pain? Pain is wise? Pain is good? What is pain anyway? Many intriguing questions to consider. Next chapter we will explore our best guesses about pain and, I hope, offer some new operating understandings and several valuable insights for us as yoga professionals. Consider this section a "trailer" for the upcoming chapter, but it also serves as an important stepping stone between the two chapters.

Suffering specifically, but pain as a related phenomenon, are among the *crucial existential issues* of our wisdom definition. The *deep insights* of wisdom require the new complex, transcontextual thinking/perceiving described earlier in this chapter. Using our fresh appreciation for adopting an intention to inquire from a relational, rather object orientation provides amazing implications for any discussion of pain. The systems thinkers have known for several decades that there is a tension between crisis and transformation that is central to the formation of complex systems.

The opioid pain crisis in the USA escalates as I am typing with almost daily revelations of corporate greed, bribes, a complicit Congress with Big Pharm, and an administration that sees opioid addiction as a moral individual failure. The gathering perfect storm of governmental dysfunction and collusion, political backwardness at best, and misguided sickcare policy present a larger organizational crisis. In systems language, these many contexts manifest as a breakdown of the existing systemic balances and at the same time represent a transition to a new state of balance. This type of crisis becomes a metaphoric "fork in the road" or, in complexity theory, what is defined as a bifurcation choice point for a complex system. Bifurcations describe choice points (right or left, so to speak) that chronologically then change the entire system beyond that point in time. The chaos of the opioid crisis with all the developing chaotic behavior, in the new scientific sense of the term, is very different from random, erratic motion. The mess of this chaotic behavior is actually deterministic and patterned, producing what are called strange attractors. Bear with me, just a bit, this is worth wading through.

Strange attractors don't develop by mere randomness, or "noise," and chaos. As emergent properties of complex systems, strange attractors create new, unpredictable creations of possibility that allow us to transform the seemingly random data/events into distinct visible shapes. One such surprise as a choice point (bifurcation) is that in the USA 2018 is an election year. The politicians know full well the electorate will be told stories about who is and isn't addressing the opioid crisis, as well as who caused it. Quite "suddenly" there is a choice point for them from what we couldn't have predicted, there is an acute interest from politicians, insurers, and the consumers for non-pharmacological pain management as alternatives to opioids. No one saw this coming or predicted these now *visible shapes* of possible opportunity for yoga therapy to be supported and possibly someday be reimbursed for pain management as a non-pharmacological option.

I offer that rather long example because it is analogous from a big picture, national perspective to what also happens when an individual finds themselves experiencing a pain crisis. They will have the chaos, the bifurcations (fork in the road of the experience choice points), and strange attractors will appear that were not available before in their tidy one, three, or five-year planners. We are literally complex systems within complex systems made up of more complex systems. Our job this section is to discuss a few more systems-related concepts that we will then be able to use to build a new understanding of both pain science and pain management in the next chapter. So, from one complex system to another, consider these fascinating pain gems.

Pain thinking: As a function of mind, cognition (thinking) in systems perspective is the activity involved in the self-generation and self-perpetuation of living networks. Basic living systems tenets are that living systems are cognitive systems, and that living as a process is a process of cognition. (That process word again from the yoga therapy and mind definitions.) The defining characteristic of an autopoietic/self-creating system is that it undergoes continual structural changes while preserving its web-like pattern of organization. Autopoiesis is more than just a gorgeous word. This self-making/sustaining property of living systems holds hope and empowerment for those we serve. Before we go there, do note that cognition is not a representation of an independently existing world (determined and the one reality) but rather a continual bringing forth/creation of a world through the process of living. The interactions of a living system with its environment are cognitive interactions (recall mutual learning), and the process of living itself is a process of cognition and therefore adaptable. A beautiful metaphor to recall this principle is to think of cognition as the breath of life. No cognition/no life.

Pain paradox of free will: While cognition is the breath of life, there are some very real constraints, however. Systems thinkers state that the behavior of a living organism is determined. Oh no, my free will, right? Hang on, as usual the explanation is both complex and nuanced with a bit of optimism buried within. Rather than the organism's behavior being determined by outside forces, it is determined by the organism's own structure. What that structure is constrains behavioral options to include cognitive potentials. The optimism appears when we remember that those very same structures formed by a succession of autonomous structural changes which reflect the mutual learning from within the environment. Change the responses, new learning for the organism, its internal systems and the learning of the environment. Hence, the behavior of the living organism is both determined and free. Now that's some paradox to sit with. Tune in next chapter to appreciate how we just described the emergence of pain, suffering, and possible ways out in the future.

Protective flinching: The natural, learned movement of the small self/ego is to protect itself to avoid being hurt again. The big Self does not need answers, it just wants meaning, and then it can live with pain. Rohr (2011, p.331) notes that "surprisingly, suffering itself often brings deep meaning to the surface to those who are suffering and also to those who love them." This flinching and the big Self's wandering search for meaning describe the dance people experiencing chronic pain find themselves tangled up in. The flinching isn't bad, but it also doesn't reflect optimal learning and cognition for the organism. Can we and our students exercise better free will options?

Viveka as a "coming soon" attraction for pain management: The yoga skill of discernment (viveka) is when seemingly good things can be recognized as sometimes bad things, and seemingly bad things can also be seen to bear some good fruit. "Yes/And" thinking, rather than simplistic either/or thinking. There is a difference between merely having correct information and the true *skillful responsiveness* of wisdom. Both knowledge and wisdom are good, but wisdom is much better. It demands a maturity of discernment, which is what it takes to develop a creative response to persistent pain. If we are frank, we must admit the vast majority of people are not there yet, and I am included in that group quite frequently. If through mutual learning we have learned to discern the real and disguised nature of both good and evil, we recognize that everything is broken and fallen, weak and poor, while still being whole and upright, strong and valuable; you and me, your country, your children, your marriage, your religion. In Chapter 4 we will explore this paradox further, but, in the meantime, sharpen your viveka and prepare your students to do the same. I'm not saying pain is good. I am saying pain is good. Is that knowledge (organized information), or is it wisdom?

Painful pause to reflect upon: Lest we get swept up into unbridled systemic optimism, consider the words of Swiss theologian Hans Urs von Balthasar toward the end of his life: "All great thought springs from a conflict between two eventual insights: (1) The wound which we find at the heart of everything is finally incurable, (2) Yet we are necessarily and still driven to try!" (in Rohr 2013, p.306). Sounds a great deal like Buddhism's First Noble Truth. This wound at the heart of life reveals itself in many ways, both as professionals and as students. Rohr once more offers a steadying perspective on what could otherwise be a deflationary prick of our bubble of enthusiasm. He offers that our holding and suffering of this tragic wound, our persistent but failed attempts to heal it, our final surrender to it, will ironically make us into a "wise and holy person" (p.306). Having lived and engaged this dance, we and our patients will become more patient, loving, hopeful, expansive, faithful, and compassionate. Now that's something to rally around. Check out the next illustration of how two prominent religious practices have choreographed dance patterns over the millennia.

WWB&JD? This "What would Buddha and Jesus do?" section is related to the earlier spiritual discussion around systems, but also a good example of how humans have addressed the dance with the *incurable wound*. Pain and suffering were the foundational teachers of transformation for both Jesus and Buddha. Respectively, that led to emphasis on compassion in Buddhist language and love in the Christian language. Buddha taught to change one's mind about what causes our suffering while Jesus taught that one should change one's very attitude toward necessary suffering, and make it into a redemptive experience for all concerned. Both recognized that pain is strong enough to gain our attention and overcome the small self's agenda. Both traditions taught in different ways, the same lesson that suffering is experienced when one is not in control. Our opposition or inner resistance to the moment produces the universal human cry of "I don't want things to be this way." Since the ego is always trying to control reality, it is invariably suffering, irritated, or unhappy, because reality is never exactly what we want. Isn't that true? Both traditions take different paths, but the transformation of the suffering leads to similar outcomes. If you haven't read any of the numerous books comparing the two traditions, I suspect you would find it both historically insightful, but also, as mentioned in the spiritual section above, a good model for shifting context for student's familial practices. Again, Rohr (2013, p.343) is such a valuable source of cross-cultural integration, sharing a quote from Lady Julian of Norwich who taught, in effect, that "there is only one suffering, and we all share in it." Sounds pretty yogic for a fourteenth-century medieval Christian mystic, doesn't it?

Wisdom Teacher Cautions

How might we recognize (re-cognition/re-think) when we aren't behaving wisely? Check yourself for the normal habits of the dualistic, not-so-wise mind: It compares, it competes, it conflicts, it conspires, it condemns, it cancels out any contrary evidence, and it then crucifies with impunity. Rohr (2011) calls it the seven Cs of delusion and the source of most violence. Without being vigilant for these habits of the dualistic mind, we will find ourselves invariably making those habits "holy," as good and necessary with a self-righteousness declaration of needing to make the world safe for democracy or to save souls for heaven, or all manner of silly, unwise declarations. Therefore, beware the Cs as you seek *accurate insight and understanding* of yourself.

In regard to interfacing with students, your local friends, and family: As you continue along the developmental path of wisdom, there can emerge a real loneliness if you are saying yes and making your wise responses and those close to you choose otherwise. Conversations may become stilted or awkward. You might find yourself no longer engaged with the old behavior patterns, and therefore change your social interactions and participation levels. Teachers counsel that you may find yourself alone more often, but also discover a new ability to be happy alone. This is solitude. Sit quietly with solitude. Rohr (2011, p.144) states this new-found preference for under-stimulation indicates you are on the "schedule of soul."

Mary Catherine Bateson (2017), noted anthropologist and daughter of two early systems thinkers, Margaret Mead and Gregory Bateson, has done a masterful job of describing a new period of life not available before for most humans. For many, there are now an extended several decades between completing family life and career progression and what used to be a brief retirement preceding a very near term death. Our increased longevity has created a new potential for what she describes as active wisdom: The enactment of our wisdom process. She cautions about the tendency to squander this unique opportunity on distractions and pleasure seeking through marketing. Instead she beautifully describes many examples of the creative responses people are making via what she describes as evolutionary clusters. These clusters are small groups of people, not necessarily retired, but intent on bringing positive, benevolent change into the world. Such processes might be a co-evolution emerging where, as individuals and collectively as a species, there are new possibilities available within the tumult of modern times. The members of those small groups feed off each other's imaginations and insights and wisdom, and then spread them out in the society going forward. Most often they are addressing either present or future suffering. Hmmm, sensing suffering, being motivated to act to alleviate that suffering, and then actually acting to do so. What a great segue into our last section. It just so happens compassion is interwoven with wisdom as the desire and motivation for the expressed benevolence that defines wisdom. Just as with yoga, pain, creativity, and wisdom, compassion is broad and complex. Let's look at some key points as they'll apply to teaching from the wisdom of pain.

Compassion

I alluded to a definition of compassion above. Compassion has been in vogue the past decade with new research and even entire departments at universities dedicated to studying it. This section will be another synopsis of some relative aspects practical for our exploration of this complex topic. Are you ready?

There are three interrelated aspects to compassion: (1) Compassion for others; (2) Compassion from others; and (3) Self-compassion (Gilbert *et al.* 2017). That relationship thing again. One's capacity to perform anyone of them is affected by the other two. There are many definitions with various nuances. We will be using this one as it is tied to the existing research while being grounded in classical terms: "a sensitivity to the suffering of self and others with a commitment to try to alleviate and prevent it" (Gilbert *et al.* 2017). Sounds a great deal like Sutra 2.16, doesn't it? (Future suffering can be prevented.)

The research has gone to great lengths to break down compassion into parts. Normally that goes against our yoga integral nature, but, for a topic as complex as compassion, parts have a large utility if we think of them as facets on the same gem of compassion. The facets of this multidimensional process include: (1) Attention to and recognition of suffering; (2) Universality and shared affective human experience of suffering or resonance; (3) An intention to relieve that suffering; (4) Motivation to respond to relieve that suffering; and (5) Affective tolerance to the uncomfortable feelings in response to the suffering. In order to be effective, one must engage and act/perform wisely. There's that wisdom stuff.

As yoga professionals, we need to be able to accurately detect the stimuli that signal suffering in ourselves and others, and also to have trained a repertoire of behaviors to fulfill our or our student's motivation. This begs the question: Can compassion be trained? I find Roshi Joan Halifax's (2012) position to be most consistent with our exploration and refer you to her brilliant article addressing that very question. The short answer is that she doesn't think compassion can be trained, but that certain practices that we'll define in Chapter 5 on creativity can prime one for the emergence of compassion. Note distinguishing the difference between training and priming for emergence of behavior, you will see it again.

Gilbert *et al.* (2017) give a detailed explanation of the many facets of compassion and their interrelationships. Significant for us is, first, that our ability to both give care and receive care drive our ability for self-compassion. If we give and receive care, then we tend to be more self-compassionate. If we only give care but don't receive well, our self-compassion suffers. This has significant implications for our sustainability in our mission. Many of the practices you will note are devoted to that self-care for this very reason. Second, there is a repeating, interwoven process in compassion where the stages/components are each rooted in skills that Halifax (2012) described and that we will highlight in Chapter 5. As a complex system, we need to appreciate the importance of the intention to be compassionate; being able to sustain attention to identify and sustain wise behavior to alleviate suffering; to establish empathy by both experiencing a similar emotional experience and being able to cognitively realize it isn't our experience; tolerance to that distress of suffering to approach rather than avoid or project our needs into the process; to maintain non-judgment around our efforts, others' response, and the ultimate outcome; to have the courage to act after reasoning, imagery, and mental rehearsal; and then act and continue the cycle moment to moment as the situation unfolds.

It helps me to hold this process in mind when I equate it to a metaphoric asana practice. We start with an intention, pay attention, deeply experience, sustain engagement, make adjustments wisely, stay with the asana, and withhold judgment, and so forth. Can you feel the cycle when you re-read the compassion asana above? I also found it helpful to draw it out on a piece of paper, letting my motor and visual systems integrate the concepts. Give it a try if you aren't feeling it yet. This is very important foundational understanding that the remainder of the book is rooted in.

The bottom line is that compassion is contextualized, à la Nora Bateson, in supportive relationships. It can only emerge if each of the facets are polished and engaged. In fact there are studies that suggest that having a sense of self that is more interdependent than independent, more complex than simple, and more fluid than fixed, leads us to greater psychological health, including greater resilience and happiness. Almost too good to be true.

There are also some much less rigorous, but heart-warming considerations around the topic of compassion to balance this more academic model. One is that all humans, to include those living with chronic pain, long to matter, especially in the lives of those whom they love. Everyone would like to believe that their existence serves a purpose. After all we are "meaning-seeking" creatures. "Only by connecting with other people and actually making a difference to others and bringing joy into their lives is it that we make our own lives matter, that we bring worth and purpose to our lives" (Jinpa 2015, p.15). Jinpa claims that this phenomenon is the power of compassion and can be summarized by the idea that "The more we are in it for other people, the more we get out of it ourselves" (p.15).

I find it fascinating that in the Buddhist tradition compassion is one of the "four immeasurables," the other three are loving kindness, sympathetic joy, and equanimity. Those are pretty easy to consider. What I find even more intriguing is their concept of both near and far enemies for each of those virtues. The far enemy, or opposite, of compassion is cruelty. That makes sense. Not so obvious to me was that the near enemy is sorrow. As I understand it, if we fail the three-sided model of compassion described earlier, sorrow can easily engulf us and prevent our being compassionate. That doesn't mean we won't experience sorrow, but, if unchecked, that emotion can derail our best efforts.

We yoga professionals deal with metaphysics by definition. Have you ever looked up what that means? Again I love words and their history. *Meta-* is a prefix, from the Greek, meaning "beyond," as in metaphysics or, literally, "beyond physics." Jinpa notes, however, that we use meta- in everyday language to mean a bigger framework within which we can describe particular phenomena we are studying. His example is "metadata is data about data, and metacognition is cognition of cognition, or thinking about thinking" (Jinpa 2015, p.107). He notes that much of what we try to develop in compassion practice is meta-awareness. We will examine why that concept is so key in our creativity chapter. Just stay aware.

His summary of the goal of compassion training is simply this: "to temper our heart and mind in such a way that we instinctively relate to ourselves and others with awareness of our needs and the basic vulnerability that unites us as humans" (2015, p.209). What a marvelous goal to balance our working model. Now, let's explore some more relationships around compassion, even a few possible downsides and cautions.

Downside of Compassion

With fame comes embellishment and overstatement. As I teased earlier about mirror neurons, even though they haven't been located in humans yet, there are books claiming they are responsible for empathy, language, even civilization. That doesn't hinder the new popular science orthodoxy's claim that mirror neurons are what make us human and empathetic. As I said, "neuro" has escaped from the laboratory and is now the wobbly foundation for considerable media hype. Standing right in the thick of it is compassion. There's some old saying about every virtue taken to its extreme becomes a vice. In an effort to illuminate the shadows around compassion as part of our accurate insight, here are some discoveries I made in my study of the topic.

There are some that argue that if we are only compassionate we are apt make unwise decisions due to resource limitations. I'm not sure I buy into that, based on the tremendous waste around so many poor choices like armaments, corporate subsidies, and the like. But within that argument there is a worthy caution for us personally that acknowledges our limitations that can lead to us having to make tough choices. Can I squeeze that last student in after a too full week? Do I participate in that book project given my other obligations that month? Do I listen to a troubled student for an extra 15 minutes after class when I'm bone tired? All questions reflecting the self-compassion component we outlined above. Thus, another balancing process of both/and, caring for self and challenging presumed constraints.

Another concern raised was a tendency to presume as yoga professionals too great an emphasis on just being compassionate. To be effective in a sustainable manner, we also need to be competent, honest, professional, and certainly respectful (O'Mahony 2017). The overlap between those skills requires awareness and reflection to keep each in a healthy balance.

There's also that syrupy, false compassion. I swear sometimes I can literally feel it. You've met the person who is empathetic without being compassionate. Compassion is not easy, because it is composed of more than just simple human kindness or false caring. Compassion also requires courage, competence, and a quality of being solid or grounded. We may be able to teach yoga professional students glib customer service skills that unfortunately come off as a superficial film of "caring-ness," but the generation of compassion in our profession will require extended priming as it can't be trained, according to Halifax (2012).

If we act "compassionately" does that mean we are sane? What is sanity? Some might say we are insane in the current milieu. Thomas Merton mused that the whole concept of sanity in a society where spiritual values have lost their meaning is itself meaningless. He wondered:

> What is the meaning of a concept of sanity that excludes love, considers it irrelevant, and destroys our capacity to love other human beings to respond to their needs and their suffering, to recognize them also as persons, to apprehend their pain as one's own? Evidently this is not necessary for "sanity" at all. (cited in Fox 2016, p.129)

Then, as the Trappist yogi he was, he wrote, "The whole idea of compassion is based on a keen awareness of the interdependence of all living beings, which are all part of one another and all involved in one another" (cited in Fox 2016, p.129). Who is crazy now? We'll return to these considerations in the creativity chapter where I will argue real creativity brings about a birth of both justice and compassion.

There is quite a great deal being written about something labeled "compassion fatigue." Both Halifax (2012) and Jinpa (2015, p.217) note that it should actually be framed more accurately as "empathy fatigue," with compassion offering a way out. Looking back at the three-part model of compassion with giving and receiving compassion, as well as self-compassion, being equal parts, failure to maintain balance isn't sustainable. Those who write of compassion fatigue are probably operating from a narrower, unidirectional definition of compassion. Practiced in all three facets it generates a self-sustaining cycle that avoids fatigue. Unbridled empathy in our pain-filled world without the appropriate self-reflection and monitoring will fatigue anyone. Beware the compassion fatigue criers.

As with the seriousness of yoga study, we are also cautioned that when studying wisdom and compassion, the topics can seem heavy and foreboding. Sages remind us to keep a playful attitude, such as in the biblical Proverbs, that describe wisdom as "delighting God day after day, ever at play in the divine presence, at play everywhere in God's world, delighting to be with the sons and daughters of the human race." Hence why I keep exhorting us to have fun here.

Did you ever consider that compassion and wisdom could be sexy, too? The topics ought not be dry, lifeless concepts. The Bible defines wisdom this way: "This is wisdom, to love life." Well, Eros is about love and passion for life, to be wise is to be erotic and vice versa. Since playfulness is part of creativity, there will be no creativity without Eros and play. Fox (2016, p.200) warns that patriarchy and capitalism fight Eros and, in the process, have reduced it to pornography. In fact all dualism makes a foe of Eros, adding to Rohr's seven Cs of dualistic thinking that we outlined earlier. Fox further noted that indigenous religion, which has been called "aboriginal Mother Love," does not despise play or Eros. And to complete this naughty, erotic blurb [sic], Rohr (2011, p.xiv) declares, "Why do I feel drawn or repelled? What we all desire and need from one another, of course, is that life energy called eros! It always draws, creates, and connects things." So by all means keep compassion and wisdom sexy in the manner of Eros.

Wisdom and compassion should also be disruptive to the status quo. Meister Eckhart says, "Compassion is where peace and justice kiss" and "compassion means justice" (cited in Fox 2016, p.240). Fox reflected that the term "compassion" is a "marriage of mysticism and justice (mysticism and passion) gives birth to the warrior energy (prophecy and justice-making), which awakens to preserve what we love and cherish" (p.240).

In completing these cautions, stay vigilant for what Rohr (2011) calls the arc of life. This arc is a common pattern of we complex individual systems. He writes clearly about what sounds like the yogic stages of life (youth, householder, and wisdom stages). He describes it as the first and second halves of life. There's broad individuality on timing, some experiencing a short first half, long second half, and others never quite getting to the second half of the arc. He's pointing to the pattern of the first half finding our way, following the rules, and being good and right. Then some calamity or what we've been calling central existential issues disrupts the first half and leads to changed behaviors, marking the second life of purpose and meaning. He advocates that if we can clarify and educate others about the common sequencing, staging, and direction of life's arc a bit more, then many practical questions and dilemmas would be resolved. The second half ideally reflects a shift from a mere survival dance to a sacred dance of meaning and purpose.

We gradually come to appreciate that these halves mimic the classic legends and literature, where the sacrifice of something to achieve something else is almost the only pattern. Wisdom and suffering stories are everywhere. The loss and renewal pattern is so constant that it can hardly be a secret. The wisdom tradition says that the pattern is and will always be true. Our final caution from noting this developmental model is that, if we try to assert wisdom before people have themselves experienced a central existential issue, we should be prepared for much resistance, denial, push-back, and verbal debate. Our service population is those with chronic pain, which means they have already met at least the existential issue of pain and suffering. There's a good chance they are ready.

A Wise Pause

Before we depart to the pain chapter all full of wisdom and compassion, I suggest we pause just a moment.

Knowing wisdom has a developmental aspect to it, there are limitations within the paradox of us being wisdom and at the same time becoming wise. Just as an acorn contains an oak tree essence, flow across time is required for that full essence to be expressed. The same can be said for our capacity to be compassionate as well. We sit in the tension of much to do now and still becoming.

How are we ever going to do both? What are we to do facing this paradox, as so often occurs in wisdom practice while also remembering that yoga is a psychospiritual practice? Rohr (2011) reminds us that all spiritual language is by necessity metaphor and symbol. The Light (wisdom) he says comes from elsewhere, not us, yet the Light is necessarily reflected through those of us still walking on the journey. He shared that Desmond Tutu reminded him, on a recent trip to Cape Town, "We are only the light bulbs, Richard, and our job is just to remain screwed in!" (Rohr 2011, p.ix).

So, keep yourself screwed in snug and here we go, let's have some fun with pain.

4

. . .

A New Understanding of Pain

MINNESOTA ADVENTURE

The source of my back pain lying there on the bed was *clearly* a bad disc. I had a postural deviation, I couldn't stand upright, pain ran down my leg, and bearing down increased my pain. Classic "bad disc," right? And what caused it? For some reason being able to point to a responsible party is an important "fact" to discover for people in pain. What then caused this calamity for me? Throwing heavy recreational vehicle tires for four summers in college? Straining my right hip helping a friend hoist the mast on his sail boat and having my foot slide out from under me on the damp deck? Landing on my left buttock when I was thrown from an all-terrain vehicle in high school? That motor vehicle accident where my legs bent the front seat ahead of me in high school? The crazy amusement park rides the day before the long drive up to the cabin? No, maybe the hot tub *after* the long drive in a flexed spine position, I'll betcha! No? Rats. We like events and isolated start points as a form of certainty for determining the source of our suffering. Twenty some years later, in retrospect I am no longer certain that labeling the precise cause is either accurate or particularly useful for serving those with persistent pain. (Note the word persistent here.) Before I share my best guess around my "cause," let's talk about what we now understand about pain. My current guess would have been the furthest thing from my list that week in the cabin.

. . .

> Compassion acknowledges the fundamental truth of our human condition that not all pain can be fixed, and that there is a limit to what each of us can do in the face of suffering. It calls for an attitude of humility. (Jinpa 2015, p.57)

So far we've deconstructed our understanding of what yoga and yoga therapy are, and the implications of that deconstruction. We have also developed a working definition of wisdom, both classical and current, and suggested the implications those definitions have for us as yoga professionals. We even hinted along the way of how those two chapters are foundational for serving those with persistent pain, to include ourselves. The stage is set. You are about to unlock the secret to vanquishing pain and suffering from the human condition. And if you believe that, trust me, there's suffering in your future. I suggest we modify our goal for this chapter to something like "Describe and discuss both classical and current understandings of pain and suffering so that you can create, with humility, new programming informed by those understandings, with the programming rooted in yoga and the wisdom traditions." I need to save the ultimate secrets for the second book to sell, don't you know?

Pain, as you well know, is another huge, complex topic. The field of pain science has been fascinating to observe the past three decades. It appears the only thing certain about pain science is that what you knew in the past has probably morphed substantially or completely by now. If I try to write about the latest understandings today, by the time you are reading this some of it will be inaccurate and new understandings will have emerged. That is how fast the field is changing. Therefore, this chapter on pain science will not attempt to nail down an absolute description as a final answer, but we will visit some general principles that have the flexibility to withstand shifting science as time unfolds new discoveries (Pearson, Prosko, and Sullivan 2019). If I am successful, you will be able to adapt your practices in line with the new facets of pain with confidence and skill as the understanding continues to morph.

One other note. Yoga therapy does not treat acute pain. There are many fine professions that do that. Remember from Chapter 1 that yoga therapy is a wellness/health science and we don't treat symptoms and pathology. We create environments for students (and ourselves) to gain insight and then wisely respond to suffering at its roots. So, from here onward, when I write pain, I mean persistent pain, not acute symptoms. While we are on the topic of acute pain, it is fun to note that the tried and true axiom of RICE (rest, ice, compression, elevation) for treating acute pain is passé now. So much for certainty.

Orientation

Last chapter we learned the Batesons' refrain that it's all patterns. This morning I awoke with an idea of how I might share the patterns within this book to orient us going into the pain chambers ahead.

Apparently during the night my systems were shepherding all of the chaos and breaking up some rigidity in how I thought this book was going to emerge. By linking some chaotic elements and freeing up other rigid roadblocks, an integration emerged.

Creativity perchance? My gunas sorting themselves out toward more balance? Divine inspiration? Integration as the fundamental human drive? Dumb luck? I certainly didn't go to bed with the intention of rewriting this part of the chapter…again. So, if "I" wasn't generating this idea, who did? Take your pick of the above explanations or offer a different one.

We need to move on to this great idea of mine. First let me offer some context for what I hope is a helpful orienteering table. Read over it with soft eyes, watch for patterns of relationship, and then just pause and let it soak in a few minutes before proceeding. I can now appreciate that this subconscious organization is also what happened in the past when I prepared for exams. I always knew when I was "ready" because the chaos would settle and a sense of barely remembering what the test was going to cover would settle in. Integration of the patterns within a skeleton of relationships was that mutual learning: "I" and the vitae changing together across time (our wisdom definition of learning).

Patterns

Vita (aspect of a living entity)	Yoga Therapy	Wisdom	Pain
Description	Complex and evolving	Complex and evolving	Complex and evolving
Static vs. Fluid	Emergent mutual learning	Emergent mutual learning	Emergent mutual learning
Spiritual	Psychospiritual	Woven through across time	Narrative, top-down component, behavior oriented
Non-harming	First yama, empowerment	Benevolent responsiveness	Self-care, SIMs, protection terminology
Focus	Health and wellbeing	Crucial existential life issues	Expanding transcontextual
Suffering	Kleshas, seeking source of suffering	Superficial and inaccurate	Kleshas, superficial, inaccurate
Goal	Prevent future suffering	Developmental benevolent responsiveness	Resilience, quality of life, relief of suffering
Epistemology (How do we come to know?)	Process of mutual learning	Process of mutual learning about self and life issues	Therapist, health team, and patient mutual learning
Certainty	Surrender and holding space	Humility and service	Open to emergence, unprestatability, "misty" (Rabey 2017)

Your Experience with Pain and Suffering

In case you don't finish this book, let's talk about what is most important first: you. I love the term "enlightened self-interest" from our aspirations of wisdom practice. All of those "mutuals" in the table above make it OK for you to admit that we're also hoping to find something in this book for you, not just those you serve. Throw away that unidirectional only serving others we debunked and consider your own pain and suffering before we immerse in the bigger topic.

Our professional interactions are a dynamic dance between our worldviews, values, needs, intuitions, expectations, and biases and those of the student, along with those of the social environment in which we both operate, and our need to feed the kids and pay the rent. However, Siegel (2017) cautions that being aware of a complex reality is one thing, but to engage with each facet of that in the most complete and honest way we can is another thing altogether. This is where the paradox of the yoga of pain being both personal and not, as well as the oneself insights of wisdom make it not only OK, but imperative, that we begin this exploration looking at us. My Minnesota thread running through each chapter is in part my execution of that principle. To not examine and contemplate our own pain and suffering leaves us vulnerable to misunderstand or project our needs in our therapeutic relationships. It also violates the three types of compassion, which then limits deep and accurate insights as well as benevolent responsiveness.

How do we do this? My suggestion is that as you read through the remainder of this chapter, you regularly pause and reflect to ask first: What in my lived BME experience can I relate this concept to? As you reflect, do any new insights emerge or deeper questions arise? Jot them down if they do. Chapter 7 on practice will give you many more ways to tease out the implications. For now, just capture them to come back to later. Then, once that reflection quiets, make the same reflection regarding those you have or are now supporting. Again, just jot them down. Nothing to fix or do yet here. Just putting light to your experience is the high value for this chapter.

It is often said that we can ignore many experiences but that pain demands an explanation. The explanations need to be deep and accurate in order to be wise. Discovering that pain perception is an output and is a best guess as to what is happening, not reality, will require wisdom and creativity. So be comfortable straddled between these two chapter themes. Because pain is an opinion on the state of one's health rather than an accurate reflection of some threat or injury, we first need to appreciate our individual biases and misperceptions if we hope to be able to create a healing environment for both ourselves and those we serve. We don't want to create further injury and pain due to unreliable assessments of each other. Therefore, as you read ahead, practice that old proverb of "Physician heal thyself" by reflecting and noting. It will save us all some future suffering.

Suffering and Pain Historical Tidbits

This section is just practical tidbits from the extensive history and exploration into these central existential issues. Part of my strategy in handling this impossible task has been to spread out the context in the opening chapters. As a refresher in the first two chapters we discussed pain as it relates to suffering from certainty; ethics and eudaimonia; ahimsâ/doing to; metaphors and pain; narrative/storytelling; Sutra 2.16; pain paradox around personal and not; futility of a certainty of pain source; separate from source; mystery of suffering; yoga as transcendence; and asmitâ versus institutional and structural suffering sources. In Chapter 3 I highlighted how pain is related to superficiality and inaccuracy; existential life issues; yearning simplicity; paradoxes; dualistic thinking; engineering systems expression; complex thinking or not; defining symmathesy; emergence; humility; death; benevolent service; complexity of the opioid crisis; pain cognition and learning; paradox of free will; protective flinching; viveka in pain management; the wound; compassion's role; and suffering and pain through religious perspectives. Gee, I snuck a great deal of pain in there, didn't I? Well please hold those many contexts as we keep mining further vitae for our mutual learning.

Seeking Meaning in Pain

Right now, you and I are seeking meaning around pain and suffering. Technically a wisdom practice if I can assume we both want to use the new meaning to respond benevolently to future suffering we encounter. Siegel (2017, p.264) offered another great mnemonic for describing how humans seek meaning: "the ABCDE's of meaning in the brain." Don't worry about the brain qualifier, we all know there is more than just brain involved, but it is the language of present day pain science that will help us communicate in wider circles. The "A" is the associations that we make from past experiences; "B" is the beliefs about life's central existential issues; the "C" is cognitions, not just superficial, but the cognitions of information flow that unfold over time to include communicating with others, about those issues; "D" is the developmental period that happens in the flow of time; "E" is the emergence of experiences that evoke emotions relevant in time and space, creating shifts in integration, not just as feelings but also changes in our state of mind. Reading this next portion will stoke your "As" and the rest of the train of relationship around meaning will unfold. Here we go.

Some Yoga Associations

For these I turn to one of my early teachers, the late Georg Feuerstein. I had the privilege to learn from Georg not only as a student in the audience, but when he and Tricia Lamb were caring for IAYT under their Yoga Research and Education Center in the late 1990s. His clarity in writing was just as apparent when I observed his dealing with future strategies around yoga and yoga therapy. Please enjoy his clarity from *The Yoga Tradition* (1998) in the form of many associative morsels about pain and suffering.

- Pain as it relates to duhkha is to the sensitive yogin the repeated drama of birth, life, and death as only pain (p.174).

- Karma leading to the experience of pleasure and pain in one of Jainism's eight primary types of karma (p.193). Jainism's attitude toward physical existence, which is experienced as a source of suffering and painful limitation (p.203).

- Giving even the slightest pain to others is to be avoided and one should strive to be helpful at all times, from the Jain *Yoga Drishti Samuccaya,* #150 (p.206).

- First Noble Truth: Life is suffering (dukkha [Pali] duhkha [Sanskrit] (p.212). Shared by Buddhism, Hinduism, and Jainism: Because everything is impermanent and does not afford us lasting happiness, our life is, in the last analysis, shot through with sorrow and pain.

- Thus we compete with ourselves and others always in search of greater happiness, comfort, fulfillment, or security, and we feel dissatisfied even in our attainments…suffering is the tension that is intrinsic to our effort to survive as separate, egoic personalities, or individuals…merely illusions…no self or anattâ/anâtman. This was a response by the Buddha to discourage the delusion that there is an immortal personal essence. He also taught that the noble truths must be deeply *felt* rather than merely *thought* about in abstract terms so that they can make their point in a student's life (*our lived BME experiences?*) (p.213).

- The second truth of desire or thirst for life (trishnâ) is the cause of suffering. Desire is anchored in ignorance (avidyâ) of our true nature, and ignorance therefore is the source of the suffering (p.213).

- Pain is an accompanying symptom of the distractions of consciousness. *Patanjali Yoga Sutra* 1.31 (p.291).

- For the discerning yogin (vivekin) the finite world of perpetual change is one of suffering, or sorrow, because change signals inevitable loss of what is desirable and gain of what is undesirable and hence unhappiness. What is to be overcome is future sorrow/ suffering. *Patanjali Yoga Sutra* 2.16 (p.295).

- Wisdom (prajna): Through the performance of the limbs of yoga, and with the dwindling of impurity [there comes about] the radiance of wisdom (jnâna), [which develops] up to the vision of discernment, *Patanjali Yoga Sutra* 2.28 (p.297).

- Kleshas the causes of affliction, *Patanjali Yoga Sutra* 2.2 (p.294). Avidyâ: ignorance; asmitâ: I-am-ness; râga: attachment; dvesha: aversion; abhinivesha: the will to live/fear of death.

Allow those to soak a bit. Is my joke about "unlocking the secret to vanquishing pain and suffering from the human condition" any funnier now? I hope the titles "pain free forever," "eliminate pain" etc., will generate a bit of light-hearted skepticism in the future. That's why, rather than trying to abolish pain, I hope to provide the groundwork for teaching wisely from our experience of pain. It's just gonna happen. Once we get to acceptance of that fact, then Sullivan *et al.*'s (2017) article about inquiring into our lived body/lived experience (LB/LE) as a body/ mind/environment (BME) points us toward discerning our samskara of habit to spark new mutual learning. That learning is the change arising from our new sankalpas via the yogic study of yamas and niyamas with implications toward our dharma/life's work. The point of such inquiry in a psychospiritual practice is to discover the spiritual driver as a causal factor or first cause, and then make incremental changes in our imperfect, humble human form. That humility includes remembering the slippery trap of asmitâ as a further source of suffering when we are ignorant of the fact that there is never a single, personally referenced cause of suffering. As much as we yearn for there to be one. While this appears to be the fuller reality, albeit a frustrating or frightening fact for some initially, the fact is that our suffering and our imperfect sense of self actually emerges from not only our inner life, but also from our inter-life as well, across unending planes of context. As complex systems, we have internal and external constraints that serve to shape our sense of self/Self and the emergence of our many experiences, to include pain and suffering. If we can loosen our grasping for a certainty around cause, are there other benefits available?

We will explore many potential benefits from that bit of hard won wisdom. Consider that our newer brain, top-down, constructed personal identity almost certainly limits our freer, more detailed, sensory-rich, bottom-up experiences of our moment-to-moment lived experience. This creates endless inaccuracies in interpreting what is taking place and decreases the quality of associations for meaning. Something new, even a traumatic injury or disease presentation, can be an invitation to attend to real time experience with essentially new lens of perception having overridden the top-down filters. But you don't need to have something that strong to begin to loosen that top-down grip. An "ordinary" experience that alters our sense of who we think we are can open us up to new ways of perceiving and experiencing life and be an opportunity for awakening. A song, a poem, or just a quiet conversation where suddenly there's the bifurcation that disrupts our system just enough and our entire BME shifts our life and identity. We breathe differently, we move in a new way, and rest at a deeper level. Can you recall such an occasion in your life? That paradox of letting go to arrive at something new that we were grasping so hard to achieve.

Avidyâ (ignorance) of our being connected has become my favorite klesha. We speak the paradox of letting go and then forget and grasp or push away. We teach unitive experience then promote our business from our forgetfulness of a commodified seller of things others need. (Like this book, Matt?) Our eco-illiteracy instead of Capra's eco-literacy. Over and over mWe fall out of right relationship to the world and to things in it and spend so much energy trying to substantiate our "reasoning" for our ignorance. Avidyâ for me has become more than mere ignorance of some data or fact, but it is misperception of relationship that appears to be the root of all hurtful behavior and suffering/dukkha, where, as Fox put it, "every movement desire tends to bear ultimate fruit in pain rather than lasting joy, in hate rather than love, in destruction rather than creation" (2016, p.175). It might be how avidyâ and our working definition of wisdom inform one another so well that is pleasing to me. Superficial and inaccurate insight leads to unskilled and non-benevolent responsiveness. That fits well for me and is a great bridge to our next section.

Some General Wisdom Associations

This section is more tidbits I mined during my research that fit nicely under a wisdom label. Now that we've established how yoga, wisdom, and pain are all evolving and interconnected, there is a bit of freedom for me to allow this section to be like that junk drawer of miscellaneous things in the kitchen. Not necessarily neat and tidy, but often where solutions can be found.

Rohr (2013) reflected how our marketing around selling comfort and ease has dislocated us from the bigger reality of unity, to include the shared existential issue of pain and suffering. We have been trained to expect satisfaction and contentment from consumption. He noted that earlier in history people lived in an inherently enchanted universe where everything belonged, including themselves despite their lot in life. And without mass and continuous marketing, people "knew" simply by listening/sensing and by observing and lived experience. They experienced what Rohr describes as the "cycles of darkness and light, of growth and death, of fertility and fecundity, which were everywhere all the time, and were their primary and natural teachers" (2013, p.131). We can certainly add pain and suffering to that list. Am I advocating a return to that time? Hardly. As my hard-working farming father in-law used to say, "The only good thing about the good old days is they're gone." We can't and I wouldn't want to return. But I think this bias Rohr highlights can sharpen our discrimination when we remember we are swimming in the marketing sea of comfort and ease that is inaccurate and superficial.

The role of memory is important for both pain and joy. Our cultural dualism will pit the two against one another as part of the marketing. Wisdom might suggest we cannot have one without the other. Again

Rohr (2013) admonishes us not to be too quick to "heal" all those bad past and present experiences unless it means we have felt them deeply and first learned what bad had to teach us. I experienced a large shift for me about *suffering* by his "ordinary" use of the word when he wrote, "God calls us to *suffer* the whole of reality, to remember the good along with the bad... Memory creates a readiness for salvation, an emptiness to receive love and a fullness to enjoy it" (2013, p.209). Suffer also means to allow, accept, endure. Suddenly my clod of *suffering* as the bad feelings around an unpleasant circumstance was broken up and woven into a deeper insight to include santosha (contentment), aparigraha (non-grasping), and ishvara pranidhana (surrendering to a higher power). A caution around too quickly wallpapering over unpleasantness is worth noting.

Carl Jung is said to have described "the legitimate pain of being human." Pain is "legit" to use the vernacular. Pain then needs to fit in our life. Failure to be with pain and learn from it is just more avidyâ, which of course leads to more suffering. If we fail to learn (that mutual thing), we almost guarantee that, rather than being transformative, that pain will help us learn a harder lesson in the future and we will probably transmit pain to others as well. It appears we are stuck needing to welcome it first and accept its legitimacy. That doesn't feel right. But I'm thinking Jung was a pretty wise guy, so duly noted.

Then I stumbled upon the three types of forbearance identified in classical Buddhist texts. Again, I'm no classical expert, so maybe this isn't as impactful on you as it was for me. The forbearances are: (1) equanimity toward those who cause us harm; (2) forbearance as voluntary acceptance of hardships in the pursuit of higher purpose; and (3) forbearance grounded in our understanding of the deeper nature of reality. There's some thinking there that flies in the face of any "real" American caricature. How do those three set with you? Reflect and make some notes if they stir anything for you. I have some work to do, especially with the first two. Although I acutely "get" the second around getting this book written.

Early in my physical therapy career I was a burn specialist and also did a great deal of general wound care. Wounding is also a key in many of our great archetypes around the existential life issues that make up wisdom. The wound can even be "sacred" (to make holy), with the

Christian story of crucifixion being the most widely known. This isn't some masochistic or sadistic spin. This is a pattern of meaning woven through much of the wisdom literature. Do you ever hear this suggested in the market place or healthcare arenas, though? Pay attention this week and take note. Why the big break from modern experience and the great archetypes?

Another bit from Fr. Rohr (2011). This nicely sets us up for our next section. The context is that he is sharing what we've all heard before around the idea that we see only what we have already decided to look for, and can't see what we are not ready or told to look for. A value of pain, suffering, failure, and humiliation is they force us to look where we would not otherwise look. That was certainly my experience in Minnesota. Self-help guides, including this book, he cautions, will help us only if they teach us to pay attention to life itself. The entire spectrum of polarities, light and shadow, love and despair, and pain and ease. It is all legit, remember. As we now plunge into the best guesses of the science of pain, consider carrying this morsel of insight from him:

> There is a strange and even wonderful communion [*yoga?*] in real human pain, actually much more than in joy, which is too often manufactured and passing. In one sense, pain's effects are not passing, and pain is less commonly manufactured. Thus it is a more honest doorway into lasting communion [*yoga?*] than even happiness. (Rohr 2011, p.158)

Follow me through the science doorway, would you?

Best Guesses about Pain

I don't intend to offend by using "guesses" instead of facts or cornerstones, or some other more permanent sounding term. "Guesses" for me is a way to keep my grasp softer and more tenuous, to avoid slipping into certainty and having to defend that certainty. I do intend, and am offering to you as well, to utilize these guesses and to stay current and adapt as the science of pain evolves. Maybe it is just my perspective as I close out my first six decades, and having seen so much change in pain science during that relatively brief period. This section begins with a very brief history of those changes and a good dose of deconstruction/destruction of what might include some "clods" of pain knowledge you and those you serve should hop on to cultivate prevention of future suffering. A review follows of the current descriptions and understandings as some pearls to consider. We will then discuss the implications of those pearls to yoga professionals, as both providers and entrepreneurs. The chapter concludes with some bridging thoughts about our responsibilities in carrying these pearls as we create our best future practices.

Bit o' History

The dominant description of pain in the twentieth century and still most prevalent today is that pain is the result of a simple signaling system. The system tracks very linearly. First some damage or insult to tissue occurs. Then nerves send an unambiguous message to the brain about the damage. The intensity of that message is directly proportionate to the severity of the injury. The brain interprets that message at face value and, if there's damage, pain is experienced at a relative level to the damage. This has also been called the light switch model. Switched on, pain is experienced. Tissue damage healed, repaired, medicated, or cut out, switch is off and no pain.

At this point, I could add three more chapters. Instead, please see the additional resources on pain science at the end of this chapter. The important point for us is: Can you see the shortcomings of that model? The collective clamor to find the offending part, fix it, and be on with it is the universal helper mantra of marketing. I know what you need, I will give it to you, and you will be pain free. Hopefully we have broken up that clod of certainty several times by now. So, if that isn't how pain is produced, what do we know now?

A short way to summarize such an answer is the story I would share with patients early in the century as our understanding was changing so quickly. Mind you, this wasn't my discovery, but what the experts in the resources list had shared. My clinic was named Dynamic Systems Rehabilitation (stealth for yoga). I invited my patients to remember that when they were having persistent pain, they should "See DSR." More specifically, the acronym CDSR. Dear patient, remember that pain is Complex, Distributed, Self-organizing, and Representational. You already knew complex was coming, right? Be wary of simplistic, certain answers. And keep in mind the contributing factors of that *complexity* are *distributed* throughout, not just within their skin and skulls, but their environments as well (that BME phenomenological thing). The self-organizing hinted at the mutual learning/changeability of their experience and it also offered hope for altering the future, but would be dependent on their claiming their agency in cooperation with their care team. The "R" invited inquiry over certainty. As just a representation of a perception of some reality, we all need to explore what our misperceptions and less than skillful and not so benevolent responses are as both provider and consumer. CDSR is quite portable and flexible. Let's unpack it just a bit more to harvest the practical pearls available to us.

What Are the Current Best Guesses about Pain?

Caution: this will be dry data dumping but a practical way to display the pearls. Pain is a multidimensional, complex experience that involves structural, sensory, cognitive, and affective factors. Chronic low back pain alone has over 200 prognostic factors (Rabey 2017). This complexity renders the treatment of chronic pain challenging and financially daunting. Further, the widespread use of opioids to treat chronic pain has created exponential growth in opioid misuse and addiction. How widespread? Chronic pain affects over 100 million Americans and 1.5 billion people worldwide and the USA spends around $635 billion per year on medical expenses and lost work productivity (Zeidan and Vago 2016). This subjective conscious experience is constructed (self-organizing) and modulated by a constellation of mutual learning to include sensory, cognitive, and affective factors, as well as mood, psychological disposition, meaning-related cognitions (e.g., suffering), desires, and pre-pain cognitive states (e.g., expectations, anxiety) all of which generates a continually changing experience across the dimension of time. The many systems feedback connections between low-level afferent and higher-order neural processes from within and amongst an environment fosters the cultivation of a *distributed*, multidimensional network associated with the subjective experience of pain. Dry, but does it help to read how pain is described in the best research? Here's some more.

The following is paraphrased from the incredible resource of Moseley and Butler (2017). Nociceptive (formerly known as pain) sensory events are first registered by peripheral primary afferent/sensory nerves (first pain, A-delta fibers; second pain, C fibers) at the site of injury/tissue damage, which then relay this nociceptive (not pain) information to the dorsal horn of the spinal cord. From the spinal cord, nociceptive information travels toward the brain on the opposite side to the brain, primarily through the spinothalamic pathway. Nociceptive input is then processed through many feedback connections between lower-level sensory regions, including the parabrachial nucleus, periaqueductal gray matter (PAG), thalamus, and primary somatosensory (SI) and secondary somatosensory (SII) cortices. Phew. Not too much more. This information coming in is then sent to the posterior and anterior insular cortices where it is calibrated to fuel the forthcoming evaluation of pain. The contextual meaning of pain is then complemented through activation of higher-order brain regions, including the anterior cingulate cortex (ACC), dorsal ACC (dACC), and prefrontal cortex (PFC). Despite being able to trace all of this signal routing, the final personal experience of pain is ultimately highly influenced by the context in which it occurs (transcontextuality anyone?). The mutual learning that includes "previous experiences, expectations, mood, conditioning, desires, sensitization/habituation, and other cognitive factors can dramatically amplify and/or attenuate pain" (Moseley and Butler 2017, pp.83–87). Fascinating material that I highly recommend exploring further. For our purposes, though, I believe I have made my point around CDSR. Can I make this material more directly applicable to our teaching from the wisdom of pain? Allow me to try.

Stringing Some Pearls

From the subset of yoga research on mindfulness-based meditation, it has repeatedly been found to significantly reduce chronic pain symptomologies and to also attenuate pain through multiple unique psychological and neural processes (Zeidan and Vago 2016). It has recently been demonstrated that mindfulness meditation is more effective in reducing pain than placebo (Zeidan et al. 2015) and can significantly alter the subjective experience of pain and fosters statistically significantly higher pain thresholds. Does this mean yoga therapy can do the same? We don't know yet, because there isn't any direct research to make those claims. What we can do is begin to articulate (pun intentional around the way the skeleton is interconnected) a rationale informed by those pearls and the following additional pearls to point toward creating practical care.

Another pearl is that pain is an output from our nervous system, not an input as detailed above. Pain is just one of many protective mechanisms we have as humans. Pain joins movement, immune function, cognition, endocrine, and autonomic responses that are all normal and necessary. Moseley and Butler (2017) note that pain is the only protective mechanism that we have a direct awareness of and therefore encourages us to do something about the unpleasant feeling. Pain can be also described as a motivator. It exists to impel us to act. When the accumulated output described above is that we are in danger (DIM: danger in me) the question becomes what should I do differently to be safe (SIM: safety in me)? Recall this is a spiritual question, based on what I believe about who and what I am, how shall I be/act? As such, can you glimpse my rationale for yoga therapy as a psychospiritual practice? One's *skillful response* presumes *accurate and deep insight and understanding* of the complex situation (read wisdom). Safety is not always possible and often the essence of the threat (real or perceived) is neither clear or escapable. This situation points us to explore the neurotag pearl to make more integrating links.

What's a neurotag? A neurotag is a term Moseley and Butler (2017) coined to describe the many outputs of the nervous system. The DIMs and SIMs above are neurotags. They aren't real objects or things, but metaphors to describe the countless outputs present moment to moment. For our context, they are a subset of Bateson's (2017) vitae, living learning complex systems "parts" of symmathesies. The relationships between the neurotags are under constant flux and reassessment, indicative of all of the learning from the change through the flow of time. Again, those two authors go into marvelous detail, but for our purposes know that they represent the changing mutual learning. The neurotags influence actions, thoughts, memories, spatial awareness, and even our unconscious "knowing." The link to our rationale is that each of these tags is not fixed in what effect they generate (uncertainty), but is modulated moment to moment by other neurotags, changing its own probability of action and response, which then changes… We saw this web of relationships in the wisdom chapter, didn't we? The significance to us is that, even though our student's description of their pain might be identical one day to the next, it is highly likely that the contributors to that pain vary not just day to day, but almost certainly moment to moment (Butler and Moseley 2017). The wisdom of Bateson's creation of symmathesy and vitae is confirmed as the best in pain science attempts to describe these latest findings, to include the neurotag metaphor. Bateson wasn't describing the experience of pain and suffering, but rather a way to hold the patterns of difference so creatively described in *Explain Pain Supercharged* (Butler and Moseley 2017). I hope this linking gives you a renewed appreciation for the importance of the level of detail we sought in the wisdom chapter.

All of this leaves us with a messy, slippery description of persistent pain experience. As pain becomes more chronic, the relationships get messier, and it sometimes loses the original connections attributed to the pain source. Said another way, chronic pain without obvious tissue damage ("Nobody can find anything") is a systemic malfunction in which the nervous system keeps producing more pain experience that is out of proportion to actual tissue damage that can be identified through testing—and sometimes this disproportion is dramatic. As Bateson warned, the mutual learning isn't necessarily beneficial or toward some higher level of development. Because the learning can go in either direction, it is more complicated, interesting, often not helpful, and in some ways, *useful* to us.

Useful? Sure. The brain decides what to make of the many inputs, how to feel about them, and what to do about them, if anything (learning). As if that didn't complicate things enough, once the brain makes a determination, it also sends information back downward that can affect the sensitivity and behavior of those nerves. This two-way learning and alteration of function is the main difference between current pain science and conventional pain teaching. Tissue damage is real and pain arising as an output from it is real. It is important not to reassure students that pain is "just" a perception and not real. We should be reassuring students that the danger implied by the neurotag may be exaggerated and that there are many biological, biomedical, and structural factors in pain in addition to the psychosocialspiritual factors already described that might also need to be addressed. We don't want to overlook or discount that important point. The pearls to share are the messiness and, as we will see later, the reason for optimism in alleviating suffering.

Students can be so discouraged because the nervous system cells that produce pain outputs get better and better at producing pain through less than ideal mutual learning. This creates a matrix mess. (Remember matrix conveys complexity and seriousness in our culture.) If students can not only hear about, but also experience how they can shift their matrix we will be headed in a good direction. That will shift them from a fixed belief around an unchangeable bad "part" to understanding that their body tissues are regulated and protected in real time by physiological events and perceptions. This includes their peripersonal space and larger environments. Friends stop calling, they are touched less often, work opportunities get limited or eliminated, mood plummets, wellness behaviors decline, rumination and catastrophization increases in a downward spiral of quality of life and dysfunctional mutual learning. No wonder students often arrive expressing what sounds like a mirror-walled crazy house of confusion, frustration, and suffering. Recall I asked early in the Preface how you would have supported me in finding my way out of my crazy house of pain? What follows are some more pearls that might reflect teaching the relationship between wisdom and pain.

Neuroplasticity Again

As promised, here are some pearls to consider around the topic of neuroplastics. First some findings, followed by possibilities for responsible application. Bear in mind as I said before, we know just enough about the topic to be uncertain about most everything we think we know about nervous systems. So humility and conservative speculation are in order in this section.

We can demonstrate that our experiences do change the activity of the brain, and that those changes can alter developing brain structure and function. The brain is dynamic and adapting, not a static tangle of wires. The brain has been shown to change in four fundamental ways as it takes in experience with the activation of neural firing. This firing, at a minimum, can lead to temporary, short-term chemical associations (learning) among neurons revealing immediate or short-term memory. But longer-term brain structure can happen even in adulthood. These changes have so far been measured in: (1) the growth of new neurons from neural stem cells, at least in the adult hippocampus; (2) the growth and modulation of synaptic connections among neurons, changing their ways of communicating with one another (more mutual learning); (3) the laying down of myelin (insulation of the nerve affecting signal transmission) by the supportive glial cells, enabling action potentials of ions flowing in and out of the neurons' membranes to stream 100 times faster and the resting or refractory period between firings to be 30 times briefer (30 x 300 = 3000 times not only faster, but more coordinated in timing and distribution) (really fast learning); and (4) the alteration of the non-DNA molecules that sit on top of the DNA called epigenetic regulators, to include histones and methyl groups. These epigenetic changes are induced by experience and then alter how future experiences will allow the genes to be expressed, proteins produced, and structural changes to unfold (Siegel 2017). All science fiction 30 years ago. Here's some more fun pearls from my Arizona neighbor, Dr. Jeffrey Kleim, PhD (2015).

Neuroplasticity was first mentioned by William James in 1887 so it's not really new, but was long forgotten. It points to neural monism (all connected/one) or, as we've discussed, the integral relationship of BME versus the old Cartesian dualism of mind and body separation. Current investigations assume that all behavior is a product of neural activity and changes in behavior can be observed as changes in neural circuits. That plasticity we did not think existed. Neuroplasticity is defined as: Any observable change in neuron structure/anatomy or function/physiology (Kleim 2015). These changes are measured by direct observation of individual neurons or inferred from measures across populations of neurons through various observational tools. Remember bifurcations in systems theory? (The forks in the road.) Well, neurons develop literal forks in the connections (synapses) as well as tree-like bifurcations on their arms (dendrites) that are called arborizations. Dendritic arborizations. Poetry in neuroscience.

There are number of factors that drive plasticity: hormones, drugs, injury, experience, disease, and electrical stimulation to name a few. More complexity and variability. And not all neuroplastics change is beneficial to the organism (hearkening back to Bateson's warning about mutual learnings). When injury, trauma, disease, autoimmune dysfunction, or other deleterious changes take place Kleim (2015) offers a great example to help appreciate the dynamism of the brain to learn during less than ideal circumstances. He uses the analogy of what must take place if, for instance, the entire violin section of the symphony went missing. The orchestra would need to write and play around the resulting gap and slowly learn to adapt back toward the behavior/sound of original score. As with the orchestra, so too in neurological rehabilitation, what is required is learning, unlearning, and relearning. The good news for us with brains is that the brain changes begin very quickly (musicians, med students, second language) in as little as months/hours.

So, to reiterate, we learned from the earlier summation of neuro-plastics changes that: All adult human behavior is skilled motor movement. Changes can begin the first day: sequence through firing pattern changes: altered gene expression: neuron structure changes: function changes: behavior changes: more gene expression changes and so on...looping in an iterative process we call life. Stuff we teachers of the transformational science of yoga really ought to know.

How might we use neuroplastics concepts? Kleim and Jones (2008) offer some guiding principles that will be reinforced in later practices. First, understand that, when we offer yoga practices, those behaviors stimulate the brain by driving synapses not specific neurons. Said another way, don't suggest you are changing specific parts of the brain. We are just offering novel experiences that may lead (see the absence of certainty?) to functional reorganization from the skilled learning that may then lead to an anatomical change (more synapses and dendritic spines). These proposed, iterative looping, entwined pathways are: behavioral signals: neural signals: plasticity: improvement of performance. Remember we don't know far more than we do know about this concept, so humility is our theme.

Kleim and Jones (2008) also offer a list of "training" principles of experience-dependent neural plasticity. Note how this interfaces with our discussion of phenomenology and the LE (lived experience) and LB (lived body) of the yamas and niyamas. Maybe those first two limbs are exercises after all? Helpful quips that could also be on T-shirts or bumper stickers:

- Use it or lose it.

- Use it and improve it.

- Specificity: Target specific skills.

- Repetition matters: Think thousands, not tens.

- Intensity matters: Goldilocks, not too much or too little.

- Time matters: Behavior close to reflection/awareness as possible.

- Salience/interest/motivation (usefulness for sustained attention… they gotta care for change).

- Age matters: But no limits.

- Transference: Shorter the leap greater the odds.

- Interference: Chronic pain, dystonia and spasticity slow the change pace.

Siegel also asked "Might the relationship between a therapist and patient also shape the brain's function and structure?" (2017, p.177). We know the quality of the relationship between the mental health therapist and client is the single most powerful predictor of outcomes. My money is on this being a crucial concept for any healing relationship and fostering the potential for neuroplastics change. Time will tell.

Emergence Some More

Can you perceive how we continue to weave back and forth between the science guesses, wisdom speculation, and yoga expressions? There's just no straight-line way to offer integral understanding. With my gratitude for your patience, we return to emergence because this system phenomenon is now being used in pain education as the grasp for certainty loosens (Rabey 2017).

Moseley and Butler ask and answer, "Can emergence be taught? Yes it can!" (2017, p.119). This is encouraging and I wholeheartedly agree on both the possibility and necessity of developing that skill. That's why we already addressed emergence as part of modern wisdom and you will discover too that many of our practices involve developing the ability to identify and allow for emergence. The authors emphasize that pain experiences as emergence are the overall best guesses from your brain about what is the most *skillful* protective *response*. A key from them for us in teaching students about emergent processes is that the student can't understand their whole pain experience just by looking at one part of it. They use a baking a cake metaphor, where you can't understand a cake by looking at the individual ingredients, as being analogous to why one can't understand pain by just looking at the joint or a single brain cell, or even just the brain. Siegel (2017) adds to the understanding when he describes one aspect of mind is that it is an emergent, self-organizing process of the complex system of embodied and relational energy and information. Note how the "S" of self-organizing from CDSR threads into "mind" from the *relational* flow of energy and information, all of which describes the *mutual learning* of the *plastic* embodied BME.

I contend we need to be able to describe emergence as science because it can very quickly come off as "magic" and fanciful without anchoring our descriptions to our culture's familiar terms. Try practicing this sequence of statements:

1. One feature of complex systems is that they have emergent properties, those qualities of the system that arise simply from the interaction of elements of the system.

2. In the case of the system of mind, the elements are energy and information. The ways these elements interact becomes apparent as time flows.

3. Where does emergence happen? Within the body as a whole, not just in the head, *and* between us: in our relationships with other people and our environment and with the world at large.

4. The intriguing name for this emergent property of complex systems is self-organization (Siegel 2017): described in CDSR.

How did that feel? No worries if a bit wobbly at first. More practice ahead. Next we turn our attention to functional uses of these many pearls for yoga therapy.

Implications for Pain Guesses to Yoga Therapy

How does one teach from the wisdom of pain? And how could yoga therapy be a creative response? My hope is you are starting to see some answers emerge. (Pun intentional and literal.) In this section I will offer some direct implications to make some of this what they used to call "lieutenant-proof" in the army when I was a lieutenant. (Do note later, though, Nora's caution around giving "direct" instructions.)

We "know," taken together, the above findings are important because they demonstrate that the neural mechanisms involved in mindfulness-based pain relief are consistent with greater processing of sensory experience and at the same time decreases in pain appraisal (Zeidan *et al.* 2015). Our familiar practices of paying attention inward and editing narratives. Pain reduction may also occur by fine-tuning the amplification of nociceptive sensory events through top-down control processes of inhibition of incoming nociceptive information and that such pain relief does not reduce pain through one avenue, but rather multiple, unique neural mechanisms. Ah, CDSR. Zeidan and Vago (2016) also cite evidence that mindfulness meditation engages mechanisms that are distinct from placebo to reduce pain and that this could be of critical importance to the millions of chronic pain sufferers seeking a fast-acting non-opioid pain therapy. See the marketing section coming up next for how to use this information. There is a decoupling between "sensory and appraisal-related brain regions," and similarly, between "sensory and affective pain" to increase coping with the pain that does improve. An alleviation of suffering even if pain is unchanged in intensity? This is the frequently reported decrease in the unpleasantness dimension of pain with respect to pain intensity (Zeidan *et al.* 2015) plus what we already discussed about yoga also altering the meaning, interpretation, and appraisal of nociceptive information, all of which could be important tools for producing more stable and long-lasting improvements in chronic pain symptoms. Wow! How do we do that?

Just a moment. First a bit more neuroplastics to fuel our imaginations. Did you know *skill* training in sensing and movement leads to reorganization of the maps (representations: the "R" in CDSR) that involve sensation and movement planning and skillful execution of *right actions*? These maps get altered with persistent pain, referred to as smudging, as though your GPS system got smeared, limiting detail and accuracy. The same skill training though can also foster "cortical synaptogenesis": birthing new synapses on the maps. More roads added to a map means more options/creative possibilities. Plus, throw in some regular endurance training when safe to begin and that can stimulate cortical angiogenesis: sprouting new blood supplies in the maps. While strength training (much further along in the progression) leads to spinal synaptogenesis: new synapses in the spinal cord. This entire cascade of neural events is evidence that skills ramp up fast but may not last; the protein responses begin the first days; synapses later around 3–7 days and maps 7–10 days. Break that pattern and no lasting change. Daily practice per Patanjali. Who knew?

There's a bit more. Plasticity only occurs if the student is paying attention. Yoga has many attention tools. The functions of movement and sensation blur together literally with parallel processes and internal parallel processing of information and the energy of signals rather than stay neatly separate. There are three full body maps in the brain and three hand maps in the primary, secondary, and supplementary movement areas. Maybe there's some systems effect to those mudras after all? Mudras haven't been studied yet, but... And there's also tremendous cross-modal (means of input/jnanendryas processing: visual/audio/tactile information and energy exchange of mind). That bodes well for a therapeutic practice that includes things like asana, chant, visual feedback, mantra, and props.

But, bad news from Nora Bateson. Do not mistake this long list of relationships with neuroplastics change with a recipe or step-by-step guide for practice. She warns that "delivery from the dilapidated state of the world now" (2017, p.189), and I add, "for the individual pain messes we encounter," is not something that can be effectively handled by a mechanic. Complex systems yoga therapy declares there are no parts to fix, so we don't need a mechanic. Therefore, there are no particular manuals to write, or scripts to edit. With spiritual challenges (this yoga is a psychospiritual practice), Rohr (2011) reminds us:

> We are the clumsy stewards of our own souls. We are charged to awaken, and much of the work of spirituality is learning how to stay out of the way of this rather natural growing and awakening. We need

to unlearn a lot… Yes, transformation is often more about unlearning than learning… (p.x)

So both we and our students will need to unlearn and mutually learn in a learning context rather than follow a recipe.

Recall we are just symmathesies within symmathesies. Our task is going to be to mine together the contexts around the pain and suffering, each of us learning and discovering the related mutual learning that takes place within our respective worlds. Think of it as though we're trying to make that presenting pain complaint "smarter" or better woven into *understanding* that is both *deep and accurate* as a wisdom process. Put another way, the pain being experienced is like an idiot light in an automotive. It means something is wrong or is in an ineffective relationship. It does not mean the person having the pain experience (the driver) is crazy, but that more learning is going to be required to get that light to change. Too often you will hear students recount the former assessment of "crazy" by others that were trying to "fix" them, rather than *learn with* them.

What do we "do" then? You may be relieved to discover that what you do will often be what you have done before, but the how and why will shift. First, however, you should have practiced and developed some mastery of whatever it is you are going to prescribe so you have more than conceptual knowledge from a book. Experiential knowledge from your own lived experience is critical in order to attune with the experience of the student, plus gain your personal insight into the suffering too. This isn't their suffering alone, remember.

Speaking of suffering, how am I supposed to *not* give you instructions while I give you instructions about how to approach all forms of pain and suffering with an open-ended yoga therapy set of skills across not just the individual issues, but institutional and societal suffering? What have I done?

My best effort to resolve this dilemma is to build another framework/skeleton of reference that will be adaptable enough to offer guidance without being prescriptive or directive, but still practical. See if this works.

- Our intention is to teach from the *wisdom of pain creatively* using *yoga therapy*.

- Wisdom requires addressing *oneself* and *others*.

- *Skillful benevolent responsiveness* is offered to self and others = *compassion*.

- There it is. What if there were a system/skeleton of organization that contained yoga therapy-type practices and supported compassionate behavior and the principles of creativity?

Roshi Joan Halifax to the rescue (2012)! Her brilliant article asking whether compassion can be trained is just such a model and I highly advise reading it. It is available free, full text on her website. The short answer to her question is that compassion cannot be trained, but compassionate behavior (action) can be primed by six practice domains of non-compassionate behaviors. This makes sense as there needs to be room to accommodate the emergence of the complex human behavior of compassion, not unlike addressing pain and suffering. Related to our next chapter on creativity, I have made a thorough argument in my textbook that this model is also robust enough to prime for another complex emergent phenomenon, creativity (Taylor 2015b). These domain practices can hold the LB/LE of all the practices of yoga therapy, to give us some organization, but also allow the dynamism of mutual learning and complexity we understand wisdom requires. Here is a list of the practices so we can have place-holders for the listing of the implications from the pain science, and please be assured we will sew/sutra them altogether in the next chapter.

Six Domain Practices

These six domain practices are tightly woven together to satisfy the demands required for wisdom as outlined last chapter (Halifax 2012; Taylor 2015b). Each informs the others, requires the others, and learns from the others. The structure is aided by placing pairs of the domain practice on an axis of relationship with another practice, leaving us with three axes. Here are the three axes with a brief explanation. The order is for convenience of memory only as they are each of equal importance:

1. *Attentional/Affective axis (A/A axis)*: The practices along this axis enhance mental balance, to include concentration, emotional regulation, and allocating mental processing resources. Our ability to direct and sustain attention on both our own and the other's (patient, student, colleague, etc.) mental state makes it possible to recognize the presence of suffering with a sustained, selective focus that is otherwise lost with misdirected (inaccurate) attention or loss of affective balance.

2. *Intentional/Insight axis (I/I axis)*: These practices of focused attention guide our mind with the intention to be compassionate that then generates insights about the suffering, the suffering's origins, and how to transform suffering in a creative emergence. These cognitive dimensions of experience interact in conjunction with the other axes. Reciprocally intention and insight also prime attention and affective balance (i.e., I intend to sustain attention on my intention to attune to my and their affect in order to gain insight...).

3. *The Embodiment/Engaged axis (E/E axis)*: We are back to LB (lived body) and LE (lived experience). What we sense, how we move, and why we move are essential to our effectiveness and our creative capacity. The science above has revealed how attention, practice, and behavior alter both function and structure of our very anatomy and physiology via neuroplasticity, epigenetic function, and the exhibition of altruistic behaviors, including compassion. This experiential E/E axis celebrates these new facts and demands our engagement (responsiveness) with all domains to prime the greatest number of emergent possibilities. We need our body and we need to act in responsiveness.

Now let's hang some practical implied practices on this skeleton to experience how responsive the model is, especially across the flow of time to represent the processes of complex symmathesies mutually learning.

Some Practices

Novelty: In order to disrupt a looping system like persistent pain, change something, almost anything, about how the person senses and feels.

Any practice beyond the habitual creates a difference (searching for the difference that makes a difference). Sensation is one of the factors used to influence pain outputs. If you can offer a practice that is small, but perceptibly different in *any way*, it may help (but especially if you can make it feel safe, protected, stabilized). The intention to pay attention to the sensation of weight bearing on the right sit bone will alter affect, require their body and engagement and may offer a new insight. Practice trying to weave all six domains with any yoga technology you might offer as novel.

Nociceptors can be nurturing: Nociception has been erroneously equated with painful inputs in the old models of pain. We now understand that the majority of nociceptive input is non-threatening and in fact can facilitate the release of factors that help tissues heal and even keep some tissues alive (Moseley and Butler 2017). A discernable but small experience of pressure, temperature, strain that can be reassessed as safe rather than automatically categorized as a danger may be the threshold into some positive adaptation. Without that shift, networks become more and more sensitive to what in fact are just safe, ordinary inputs. Specific training in these techniques is available in the resources section and is best done in person. In my experience, tempered and gentle "playing" with modest, novel inputs has been safe and well accepted by students. Just watch your ego and projection, erring toward ahimsâ. The nervous system is so sensitive, tiny changes are the rule and are generally well tolerated.

Fix what is fixable: Prioritize with the student which of the many factors identified as *insights* that are contributing to their suffering can be fixed. The new discovery by them that possibly many of the oldest problems are contributing, places the response-ability on them to apply a more skillful response toward remedying the situation instead of avoiding or tolerating them anymore. Bad marriages and toxic friendships, soulless jobs and nasty bosses, insomnia, depression, and many more will require hard work and often bringing in appropriate expertise to their team. But, now that they know, wisdom declares that more accurate and deep insight be given a more *skillful response/engagement*. Taking right action to address such problems is a direct route to easing the outputs of interpretations of pain. Avoidance insures future suffering.

Mind your scope of practice: Here's that *oneself*-ness part of wisdom. Celebrate working with a team and operating within your scope of practice. Maintaining this *intention*, noting your *affect,* and paying *attention* through your *embodiment* as you *engage* in the teaching is essential to avoid projection of your needs and insecurities around professional boundaries. A miscue in this regard can disempower the student and send the relationship careening into unintended himsâ/harming. Yoga therapists and teachers don't diagnose, don't treat symptoms or pathology, and we are not marital, vocational, or rehabilitation professionals. Stop it if you do, and stay alert as you engage to not start.

Asana-less ethics and identity: If we weave back to the first yoga chapter about identity and BME of first-person ethical review as yamas and niyamas study, you can sense how important it is to support students beyond an asana-focused approach. Recall the challenges in identity include the *affective and cognitive* experiences of the body as alien, powerless, and isolated. Such rejection from the affected body part begins an unraveling of identity with a host of challenges to include disorientation, uncertainty, loss of familiarity with their *body*, and an inability to *engage* with the world as they had before due to an altered sense of identity. Lacking a harmony within the BME and experiencing an absence of eudaimonia will require redefining the many relationships in the complexities of chronic pain. How can you introduce yamas and niyamas within the framework of the domain practices? Might take some creativity, right?

Gunas juggling: With every practice, recall Siegel's (2017) "gunas-like" definition of integration/chaos/rigidity from Chapter 2. Can you create a split attention for them to not just linking, but differentiating each practice? Optimal self-organization occurs when the system has two interactive processes occur. One is differentiating elements of the system (breaking up rigidity/tamas), allowing the experiences to become unique and have their own integrity; the other is linking what appeared to be separate elements of the system (organizing the chaos/ragas). The common modern term we can use for this linkage of differentiated parts is integration (sattva). Integration enables optimal self-organization so that a system functions with flexibility, adaptability, coherence (a term meaning holding together as a whole, having resilience), energy, and stability or Siegel's (2017) FACES. In our teaching, two individuals can also become linked as one *connected* system when each other's subjective experience is *attended* to, respected, and shared. That requires an intention to attend to feeling felt both between and within. How would you create that with asana? Pranayama? Mudra? You can. Give it a try.

Ahimsâ: Our *intention* to sustain *attention* to *engaging* in ahimsâ overrides all practices. Can you generate and sustain openness, observation, and objectivity presence? When we set such an *intention*, that creates safety and predictability for the student to enable the flow of energy and information to move toward integration. Doing to or harming does the opposite. Our sustained observation and objectivity sorting mine/theirs creates a means of detecting chaos and rigidity so that the flow can be directed toward differentiation and linkage. Because integration is a natural drive of a complex system, sometimes what we need to do is simply get out of our own way by not doing to and let integration naturally emerge. "Presence is the portal for integration" (Siegel 2017, p.281). *Skillful benevolent responsiveness.* But don't forget the *oneself* part needs to come first. Hold in mind that violence to self includes anytime you make yourself sick or dysfunctional by being overworked or carrying too much stress (a DIM in you). How you show up affects your wisdom practice, as well as the SIM for both you and your student. The first yama begins in the mirror. Our first step in a non-recipe.

Forgiveness and anger issues: Bateson (2017) cautions against the pop principles around forgiveness and anger, to include "moving on" or "getting over it." The *affective attention* for *insight* and informed *engagement* may be derailed if the ecological process of discovery is avoided within the ecology of pain. She notes that it is "anger whose fire burns away numbness" (p.148). How can you most effectively ease the numbness? Your knowing your skill level and the limits of scope of practice is essential here. Developing a healthy referral relationship with an expert is both good business and ahimsâ. Better to make the referral and turn your lens inward on your own challenges with forgiveness and anger within the domains of practice. There are many related practices in the practices chapter to explore. *Oneself* first = wisdom.

Gripping and bracing: These behaviors can be both literal and figurative. DIM assessments generate the desire to hold one part of a system still in hopes of safety (a form of the complex freeze, flee, and fight responses). To brace either way requires that all the relationships upon which this braced area is interdependent must be altered to absorb the holding as every other interaction within the system must compensate for the lack of "flexibility" in one part. This security plan is temporary at best. Before long the larger patterns of the system will overtake an attempt to keep non-changing in place. The much larger ecology of their systems will continue. The intention to brace the pain area will alter the breathing pattern, that changes the autonomic nervous system state, leading to a different affect with a potentially inaccurate insight around DIM, diminishing resiliency for additional loads, building chaos despite the rigidity, and on and on. Can you sense those loops and weaves? Might you offer practices that allow sensing (*affect*) via *attention* for *insight* through the *embodied* experience for new *engagement* strategies? Fascinating how *wisdom* leads to *practice domains* to enhance *wisdom* via *yoga therapy*, isn't it?

Don't… Oops, that is a directive… An implication from Bateson's (2017, p.149) systems science regarding "direct correctives" to systems problems include "our children, the ecology, the economy, etc." Pay careful attention in your teaching to how often you direct rather than invite consideration or exploration. Those directives are your power grabs. Systems science suggests that diffused adjustments are more effective in complex systems and indirect is much more effective, though impossible to prescribe. Rats: Impossible? She states:

> The paradox of order and chaos in simultaneous improvisation is such a challenge to hold in focus. But in that balancing (for it is surely in infinite process and never totally balanced), in that conversation, in that music, the new enters the patterns. (2017, p.149)

Can we sustain the intention to invite rather than direct? You are hereby invited.

Pain yoga therapy rules: Now that we have that "no directives" out of the way (a joke), here are some handy rules to carry with you. The paradox of no rules need rules.

- Get people moving with a sense of control and safety (SIM).

- Co-author a convincing story together about the experiences using the above pearls on a wisdom trek.

- Instruct yoga technologies in context with that story.

- Provide novel inputs, avoiding excessive repetition of any single input.

- Meet their expectations around control, comfort, and a sense of safety.

- Build self-confidence and restore self-efficacy/trust in their LB and LE.

- Listen and really hear what they report during sessions and from their discoveries at home.

- Follow the person's interests and values, not your agenda. Goals are the student's, not ours.

- Be with rather than do to.

- Admit you don't know often, but celebrate the future mutual learning that not knowing invites and the mutual discoveries ahead as you both engage further in the process.

As I mentioned, Chapter 7 contains many more domain practices by domain, but also by each chapter's theme. These were just the highlights and a basic frame of reference to begin creation. Speaking of creation, the words you use in marketing what you do as a yoga professional are often the first "touch" between the symmathesies of you and the student. That means your words deserve a great deal of *attention* in order not to inadvertently add to the suffering.

The Marketing Talk

We have spent a great deal of time describing and building language around yoga, wisdom, and pain. The narrative or stories we humans tell one another drive our top-down editing and sense of safety (SIM). From your first conversation with them or their first read of your marketing material, there's a story being edited. We know that for millennia a sacred myth can keep a group of people healthy, happy, and whole, even inside their pain both individually and collectively. Good stories give deep meaning, and pull us into what O'Donohue (2017) calls "deep time" (which encompasses all time, past and future, geological and cosmological, and not just our little time or culture). How we build such stories can become the very food that sustains us, and the well-edited story points us toward what we are trying to get back to, which is often home and safety in the fullest sense. Mary Catherine Bateson (2017) shared how important creating an environment in which learning is possible is to give a sense of home. "And that is what a home is. I mean that is what we want the homes that we give to our children to be—places where they grow in many, many different ways." If our students in pain can learn how to connect with other people and how to care for others within their story, this builds a home feel. In a home environment, they learn their own capacities and how to trust their body, other people and how to trust themselves. A good home environment allows human beings to remain playful, and play is a very important part of learning and experimenting. Mary Bateson (2017) notes that "most other species, they figure out how to be a rabbit or a chicken or an owl or a fish, and that's what they do for the rest of their life; so learning is us." This quality storytelling and home environment (both within and without) isn't new. O'Donohue shared that, at the end of Latin prayers, it would be written, "Per omnia saecula saeculorum," loosely translated as "through all the ages of ages." Keep this in mind as you review the following ways you can begin to build a new story and home from your first conversation or marketing text through the deepest, most intimate yoga therapy sessions. The story is always unfolding. Let's craft a healing one grounded in a safe home again, or for the first time.

Sell hope but shoot straight: I would love to have a dollar for every time a student completed a phone inquiry or their initial history and then asked, "Is there hope?" The answer is nearly always the same: yes, there's hope. There's *never* a guarantee, but there's *always* hope, and recovery from most kinds of severe chronic pain is not only possible, but happens fairly often. Which, of course, also means it doesn't happen fairly often too, remember. As a guideline, with some rare exceptions, there need never be any reason to fear that improvement in *suffering* from any chronic pain problem is impossible. We can share that for the same reasons that pain can be ridiculously stubborn and out of proportion to any obvious cause because of its complexity, so to the suffering also never rarely loses the potential to finally shift and improve. Keep this clarity in mind because yoga therapy is about wellbeing and health, not curing and pathology.

Safety reigns: The potential student is experiencing DIMs. Safety is what they seek, even if they can only verbalize it as pain relief. Emphasize safety in all regards. Not overselling. Emphasize how yoga therapy is non-violent and empowering. Educate that pain is the end result, and as an output of the brain designed to protect them not harm them. The goal of your instruction will be to teach them how to be kind to their nervous system. Together you will teach them to be able to create pleasant, safe sensory experiences. These positive inputs increase comfort and a sense of safety and rebuild trust in their experience of their body. In order for them to reduce their pain and suffering, together you will create ways to offer good evidence of safety and discredit what to date has signaled danger.

Surrender, me? Be honest and acknowledge that learning acceptance that pain is a part of being human is a goal. That doesn't mean together you won't exhaust every avenue to reduce pain. Your humility and willingness to acknowledge that there may always be some pain will be a breath of fresh air. It is also at this point you can test the waters of yoga therapy as a spiritual practice as well. Sharing the niyama of ishvara pranidhana (surrender to a higher power) does not mean giving up. Surrender means turning over authority to, not quitting. Such a metaphorical emptying out is only for the sake of a potential outpouring into the space created by surrender. Ishvara (as it means to them) is like nature and nature abhors a vacuum. Into that blank canvas can flow transformation, healing, and a new identity that we can't predict today, but only if space is available and that space happens in surrender. Tell the story of every great hero archetype, with the student as the heroine/hero. It matters and for most students, will require a huge edit.

Pain is not "all in your head": This is the most common misconception when people are told the pain science story. There are a few people for whom this is true and the condition is hypochondria, a form of anxiety disorder, a mental illness. That's *not* what we are implying. What we mean is the output of what they experience as pain is their system's best *guess* to keep them safe, but can be mistaken like any other assessment they make. Sharing all the sources that *guess* is based on can help them appreciate what a complex job the system has. Saying something like:

> Did you realize your system sits around a board table with the following departments making often wildly different reports? The departments are roughly: Beliefs and meanings 13 percent; Survival valuing 10 percent; Fear avoidance 10 percent; Catastrophe creators 13 percent; The sleep deprived 19 percent; Stress and anxiety 16 percent; Depression 10 percent; and Nociception receiving department 10 percent. Isn't it amazing this boardroom ever comes up with an accurate assessment? Our job will be to step in as consultants and address every one of those departments to improve management decisions. Will you join me?

Our new yoga definition offers consultants for each of those departments.

Brain personnel management: When you share your story by describing the known benefits of yoga practice as they apply to the different departments of that brain board meeting it will be news to them and intriguing. You will be describing the prefrontal cortex anatomy, but avoid using these anatomical terms and just note what the research says about how yoga practices can shape up these departments. The functions addressed include: (1) body regulation (balancing the body's brakes and accelerators); (2) attuned communication with self and others (focusing attention on their internal mental life); (3) emotional balance (living with a richer inner experience of feelings); (4) response flexibility (being able to pause in a space before responding); (5) soothing fear (calming fear reactions/SIM); (6) insight (connecting past, present, and future with more accurate self-understanding); (7) empathy (sensing the inner mental life of another); (8) morality (thinking and behaving as part of a larger whole, broader than a personal, bodily self); and (9) intuition (awareness of the utility of the input from the body). There are many more and collecting them can be very useful for this communication process. Keep it simple, but informed by research, not speculation. And they don't have to believe you, because they will confirm it through their direct experience of the practices. Sell these benefits you offer to them, not the features of your training or lineage.

Pain management, oxymoron? George Carlin would have had fun with this one. Humor can be a good way into a deeper storytelling. Pain and suffering is complex, and needs a parallel complexity of care to meet it. That is what separates yoga therapy from other therapies. Sure, we wish for an easier way out, or to provide some vanishing trick to the person or institution that is suffering. Normally, though, it is going to require a robust practice that can match the complexity. And if the source of the pain seems to come from another person, that's OK and in fact means they still care rather than having gone completely numb. Caring is good. Reassure them that caring enables one to learn, even when resentment can feel too difficult to sustain. Learning means we can heal and evolve, à la our chapter on wisdom. In fact, as we explore in the pain pearls, usually the learning itself (higher order organization) is a moment at which the pain is not healed so much as it appears to become obsolete. Given our oxymoron, we can assume the pain is not locatable in a particular vein of thought, body part, or aspect of being, but rather that it is distributed everywhere. Good luck managing.

Where are da' guys? This is a question that bears consideration as we craft our conversations. This spot here seems as good a place as any to post it. Why so few men accessing yoga? That's a symptom we do need to address in our storytelling. Rohr (2011) noted, when discussing who adopts non-dual approaches, that men are actually encouraged to deny their shadow self in any competitive society. Ever the strong and hero, vulnerability is weakness, etc. His observation is that all we end up with are a lot of sad and angry old men. Any male readers out there? How are you going to structure your conversations and practices to address this symptom of society? Can we heal with only primarily one gender participating? Another complex, unsolvable question I know. Keep it mind though when choosing your stories and images to support those stories. Does what you are posting or saying allow everyone to feel comfortable here, even we little boys trying to be superheroes?

How did I get here? A common query to all of us from our students, isn't it? How we help them build their answer is key. The yoga developmental story can support that process: youth; householder; wisdom years; and withdrawal to death. An arc of life. Not fixed to any particular age per se. Our first tasks in youth and householder periods we usually take for granted as the very purpose of life: career, relationships, and survival. The second half of tasks of discovering meaning and wholeness Rohr says is more encountered than sought. We are back to yoga as a psychospiritual practice. Our students, and us, arrive at these second half of life tasks without much preplanning, purpose, or passion (Rohr 2011). In our self-help culture encounters with challenges such as pain and suffering are things to be surmounted and eradicated, ever onward and upward. Rohr offers that the sacred wound of such encounters teaches a most counterintuitive thing: "that we must go down before we even know what up is" (2011, p.275). What he offers for me is a difficult teaching. He contends that suffering seems to be required in order to destabilize both our arrogance and ignorance. We *will be* wounded, as we read from the yoga texts at the beginning of this chapter. Our suffering is potentially redemptive, especially if through practice we discover what about our suffering can transform our story to include being a sacred wound (as a part of the meaning, not the entire meaning). The practices we offer form the container where the student's innate wisdom can manifest in deep and accurate insight. If there isn't some way to find deeper meaning in their suffering, people will normally close up and close down. Tread wisely in your serving those that ask this question. We don't have the answers, but rather offer the support and space for them to create their own. This falling down to go up of Rohr's is another tricky integral paradox.

Humility again: The root of humility is humus: earth. That's the stuff we can touch (or at least believe we are touching, for the purists). There's a meme that reads: Relax, nothing is under control. There is a form of freedom hidden in that meme. A question requiring humility is "What is healing and how does it happen?" I share Bateson's premise that the idea of mutual learning between and within living contexts is where healing can happen. And that learning does not stop. Nor will the learning always be progressive or good. Many times the learning will be in a context that includes pain, addiction, pathology, and so on. There is no controlling mutual learning. Mutual learning cannot be "solved." With our earthiness, we can only become more able "to take in and consider the complexity we are faced with if we approach it from this stance" (2017, p.140). No surety, just humility. That feels like deep and accurate insight to me. How about you?

There's no place like home: In our various searches for SIMs, there is often a component of the archetype of longing for return or getting *home* (in the individual's best sense of that word because their *home* wasn't necessarily equated with safety). Now put this powerful myth in the back of your mind as we dive into this exciting exploration of the further journey. It can operate as a sort of blueprint for what we want to say if together you and they discover what home would be for them. What you create together won't be a static house, but the whole story will be set in the matrix of seeking to find *home*, then leave from home, and then to return there. Life is a process of refining and defining what *home* really is. The goal in sacred storytelling is always to come back home, after getting the protagonist/student to leave home in the first place. Our practice is to discover how home has a whole new meaning, one they might never have imagined before. Yoga, being a transformative practice, means the new meaning will transcend, but include, their initial experience of home. Another yoga polarity dance. Rohr describes it as, "We are both driven and called forward by a kind of deep homesickness, it seems" (2011, p.89). The polarity is a dissatisfaction that both sends out and calls us back. He points us back to our yoga as union with the divine by suggesting that *home* is another word for the Spirit that we are, our True Self. Finding ourselves in another paradox of that self-same moment that we experience the divine in ourselves, we also find ourselves inside the divine. A homecoming, if you will. When our teaching has been effective, there will also be an insight discovered that homes are not meant to be lived in, but only to be moved out from. Such a tangle of complexity.

How are we going to create such environments for ourselves and our students? Living with chronic pain can seem to be experienced as falling downward into an abyss. To use Rohr's terminology, paraphrasing, what can in fact happen is that the person may fall upward and onward, into a broader and deeper world, where they find their fullness, finally connected to the whole, and now can live inside the Big Picture. To arrive there is going to require creativity.

Creativity Ahead

Beware the temptation to build an edifice of certainty with all this incredible science of pain. Science is after all a best guess at best by its own admission. Sure, there are those that have made a religion out of it, but wisdom cautions us via the three humilities to be care-full. I have very deliberately constructed this book to not be a, "Here's all the shiny new parts, assemble and align them like so, and you will be doing things right" fashion. I don't know what such a manual would look like and you don't either. That includes all of us.

O'Donohue (2017) spoke of thresholds very elegantly. Perhaps if we think of this final section of this chapter as a threshold from a world seeking certainty back through a forest of beauty and mystery that will put us in a more appropriate frame of mind and heart. Our expression of wisdom is indeed to "thresh" (separate valuable from not necessary). The metaphor of stepping from one amazing room into another equally amazing room contains the movement of development as part of wisdom. Allow me to highlight the following many specimens of this mysterious forest to enchant and engage your transition toward our next chapter.

"*Beauty* isn't all about just nice loveliness," said O'Donohue (2017). Beauty should also be about a more rounded, substantial becoming in our life. In this forest, reclaiming the beauty of our life and that of our students is the quest. He noted that when life has us cross a new threshold, and if we cross the threshold worthily (wisely?), that there we may discover and heal the patterns of repetition that were in us that had us caught somewhere (samskaras). What if the person in pain standing in a threshold could cross onto new ground, where they no longer repeat what they've been through in the last place they were? Sounds like the beauty of yoga, doesn't it? Our task coming out of this wood will be to create a practice where *beauty* emerges within the pain, and is about an emergent fullness. Done wisely, there ought to be "a greater sense of grace and elegance, a deeper sense of depth, and also a kind of homecoming for the enriched memory of their [our] unfolding life?" (O'Donohue 2017).

Perfectionism: True confessions from a recovering valedictorian. I suspect a few of you can also relate to this species. The Tibetans encapsulated the problems with *perfectionistic* self-esteem in the memorable saying "Envy toward the above, competitiveness toward the equal, and contempt toward the lower" (Jinpa 2015, p.31). Might these attitudes be at the root of our and our students' dissatisfaction and unhappiness? *Perfectionism* is a fine specimen for reflecting our self-kindness. That quality of self-kindness is one of Neff's three components of self-compassion (2011). Common humanity and mindfulness being the other two components.

Examining our self-kindness reveals how we view our shortcomings and difficulties with kindness, understanding, and acceptance versus negative judgments. Clothed in the three humilities, we have permission to allow this species to be, but we should revisit from time to time if it is part of our pattern. *Perfectionism* keeps us from accurately feeling connected to ourselves and of course to others too. If perfectionism were actually a part of the flora, we would probably label it a weed, but not one to ignore.

The next species is the joy of *awareness of awareness*. One of the many fruits of practice is direct experience of being aware of our awareness. Can you remember the first time you came across this species? We must not lose the newness of that experience. For within it lies a pointer on the path to wisdom. The silence, the awe, and the space around *awareness of awareness* could easily be described as sacred. Cultivating this fruit for ourselves gives new ways to create experiences that allow those we serve to enjoy it as well. The silence of a deep woods is a powerful metaphor for describing this beauty. Tread quietly.

The constant problem: The gardeners and lawn keepers that are reading surely have a pesky specimen, whether flora or fauna, in their role. Around suffering we can also appreciate that the suffering itself does not solve a problem directly so much as it reveals that we are the *constant problem* to ourselves (Rohr 2011). Just identifying this species can open up new spaces within us for mutual learning and reinforces the importance of *oneself* in our wisdom definition. Stop looking outside ourselves for the solution and kindly tend the constant problem that is us. In a self-kindness kind of way of course.

Our stories are often constructed of the most banal, secondhand psychological and spiritual cliché, and we look at a student's beautiful, interesting face telling a *story* that we frequently know doesn't hold a candle to the life that's secretly in there. We constantly reduce our identity to biography, exacerbated by social media. O'Donohue (2017) stated they're not the same thing. He believes biography unfolds identity and makes it visible and puts the mirror of it out there, but that identity is a more complex thing. He pointed to fourteenth-century German mystic Meister Eckhart's quote, "There is a place in the soul that neither time nor space nor no created thing can touch." What this means is that our identity is not equivalent to our biography and that there is a place in us where we have never been wounded, where there is still a sureness in us, where there's a seamlessness in us, and where there is a confidence and tranquility in us. From his description, I think that the intention of prayer and spirituality and love is now and again to visit that inner kind of sanctuary our stories can hold for us. In this realization, we are reminded of the unmoved Self of yoga. Tend your and their *stories* with great care to nurture *stories* that contain these important seeds of Self.

Utility: Jinpa (2015) noted that the most compelling thing about compassion and kindness is the way they bring purpose to our life. Another word for purpose is *utility*. I still remember resonating with Michael Caine in the movie *Cider House Rules* when he declared his purpose in life was to be *useful*. I think many of us share this longing. Jinpa concluded, "There is nothing like the feeling of being *useful*" (2015, p.16). We discover this same species of utility is the centerpiece of what defines creativity as well. Now that's useful.

The Flytrap: As a child Venus *flytraps* fascinated me. Are they plant or animal? The way they allured the flies through light and scent. Their slow, insidious embrace of the fly that went unnoticed until too late. Probably not very yogic of me to not have compassion for the fly, in hindsight? As we approach creativity, do note that our *flytrap* is our chasing the sea of endless books and teachers for the solutions to easing suffering. Just one more book (after this one), one more workshop or business development course, and then I will create. And repeat, over and over as the *flytrap* holds us in its embrace, sucking our unique contribution as a creator out of us. Suddenly months and years have passed and we haven't noticed the stickiness of our *flytrap*. It is time to take flight and seize our freedom of *being* creativity (very different from *being* creative, mind you, another trap). *Flytraps* end up full of desiccated, lifeless fly-bits that even they disgorge. We are meant for something more.

Mystery: Carl Jung wrote, "Life is a luminous pause between two great *mysteries*, which themselves are one" (Jung 1980, p.483). We all walk through life with its *mysteries* (central existential life issues?) wearing many masks. The masks are not bad, evil, or necessarily even egocentric. They just are not "true." In order to deal with the *mysteries*, we manufacture and sustain many masks in our masquerade. For we yoga professionals, this is especially sensitive as it makes us into hypocrites on some level. Hypocrite has its origins in Greek, meaning "actor" or someone playing a role rather than being genuine. We see this in the yoga community regularly, as well as in ourselves. Why are purveyors of realization hiding behind masks to avoid the *mysteries*? The black and white, dark and light of thespian masks hearken to what John of the Cross called "luminous darkness," when musing about life's *mysteries*. Stepping up to be creativity will require that we experience the simultaneous co-existence of deep suffering and intense joy. Rohr reminds us that early in life's first half (before we meet face to face with the deep existential life issues), it is probably necessary to try to eliminate most doubt as a good survival technique. But he rightly acknowledges that such a worldview is neither true or wise. Wisdom, he noted "happily lives with mystery, doubt, and 'unknowing,' and in such living, ironically resolves that very *mystery* to some degree. I have never figured out why unknowing becomes another kind of knowing, but it surely seems to be" (Rohr 2011, p.112). And how about this for possibly the best botanical Latin name we might apply to *mystery*? *Docta ignorantia* (learned ignorance). This ignorance isn't that of avidyâ, but the realization of the humilities of wisdom. So cut a big bouquet of *mystery* to take along. We are off to creativity after a short stop in Minnesota.

MINNESOTA ADVENTURE (CONT'D)

Now about that "bad" disc of mine? As a form of review, let's list my assumptions and what this chapter says about my assumptions.

Assumptions:

- *There was a single source of tissue damage creating the pain.* While there often is an accident or trauma that is abrupt, the tissue doesn't take 10 years to heal. Something else is going on.

- *I had a bad disc.* First, does a lumbar disc have the capacity to be "bad" of its own volition? No. Does it exist in isolation? No, it's part of all of me and woven into not just my anatomy, but influenced by my psychosocialspiritual status as well. When someone describes a part of them as "other" than themselves, that is language that points to a disembodiment from that part/vita of them. That calls for an integrating edit of that narrative.

- *A long list of prohibitions and admonitions for what to do and avoid doing will lead to resolution of the pain.* Well, if pain is an emergent process from a complex living system to include the individual, their environment, and their culture, how can such list ever possibly address all the factors, since the condition isn't predictable in the first place? (More on this in the next chapter.) Quite simply there is no such list and there can't be. General guidelines can be supportive, but those emphasizing one's capacities, opportunities, and encouraging full function appear to be important (Moseley and Butler 2017). A stark contrast from my "don't bend forward," "don't slump sit," "do lots of unnatural back bends all day," "avoid lifting," "be careful!," and so on.

- *With a damaged disc the best I could hope for was not to make it worse and hope later life arthritic changes would stabilize the disc dynamics by essentially rusting it in place.* Well, there's another messed-up narrative. Now we know herniated discs can heal and that they literally do not "slip." How did I ever get better with those stories I told myself?

- *Bad back pain like this was the result of psychospiritual issues. Ha-ha, right! Or so I would have thought. It is a disc, what do mind, emotions, or spirituality have to do with it causing me pain?*

. . .

What was the source of my pain then? Well, if I tell you now, you might not read the next chapter! I promise, I'll give you my best guess there. For now, consider your and your students' stories about their pain. Does anybody's narrative need a good, thorough editing after absorbing this chapter's information? How, then, are we going to be with each other in pain? Grab that big bouquet of *docta ignorantia* and let's go find out.

The Changing Pain Landscape of Resources

The world is full of pain resources. Some good. Some very bad. The following are by leading authorities with good reputations.

Free Online Course

Try the free patient education program at the Retrain Pain Foundation: www.retrainpain.org.

Videos

Lorimer Moseley, *Why Things Hurt*, TEDxAdelaide, featuring Dr. Lorimer Moseley with good science, great storytelling and humor: https://youtu.be/gwd-wLdIHjs.

Greg Lehman, *Back Extension Hinge Is Not A Flaw*, featuring Greg Lehman, PT, DC, and professor of biomechanics who makes the complex more understandable: https://youtu.be/K6b4rwydAis.

Books

The *Explain Pain* books by Butler and Moseley are excellent. Seminars available as well: www.noigroup.com/en/Store.

Blogs/Websites

Neuro Orthopedic Institute: https://noijam.com

Bronnie Thompson: https://healthskills.wordpress.com

Lorimer, Mosely, & Co.: https://bodyinmind.org

Diane Jacobs: http://humanantigravitysuit.blogspot.co.uk

Neil Pearson, PT: http://lifeisnow.ca

Greg Lehman, PT, DC: www.greglehman.ca

5

. . .

Creativity: You've Got This

MINNESOTA ADVENTURE

We human beings are such marvelous storytellers. The drive to make our experiences make sense is so strong. There was a real battle of stories going on in my mind that week in Minnesota to both understand and find the "why" for what I was experiencing. A major infestation of *docta ignorantia* around the cabin that I couldn't even see. Included in those many stories were, of course, some from the past, but also projections into the future about what lay ahead and how it would all turn out. Constant editing, future, past, future, and back, but not much on the present. The parts guy didn't yet appreciate the power of calming my nervous system, nor did I have any skills to relax other than to take a very long run to exhaust myself...and that wasn't going to happen.

I did realize I needed to change or adapt some things as the current course was not working for me. This urge, as we just read, was my innate state of *being creativity* itself, rather than my inaccurate conclusion that I needed to be *thinking creatively*. This misidentification of self (non-realization?) literally gave me a form of writer's block in my own stories. Added to my training and worldview ignorantia, any talk of emergent properties of complex living systems would have been dismissed as magical thinking or New Age baloney. I *knew*: Find all the parts, line them up in different configurations, and then things would work—literally. Line my spine up, move in certain ways and not in others, then my pain would be gone. Funny how right now I can see what a much deeper metaphor there was in that approach.

. . .

The depth of that metaphor of controlling all the parts and thinking that would achieve predictability (aka safety) sure seems silly today. But still, even now, I find myself re-editing that storyline to make the experiences make sense. Only now I say things like:

> Oh, I was in a sympathetic state all of the time, trying to be good and then safe, but that made me breathe from my chest and not my diaphragm, which meant I had very little postural stability from limited intra-abdominal pressure, which was deviating my posture and creating the disc herniation and once I learned to breathe and relax, that stabilized my spine making my bad disc good, and then I started letting go of trying to control every part of my life which allowed my brain to function beyond a lower cortical level survival mode, and actually fire at a higher level in the layers of the neo-cortex with other associated centers to *create* new insights that then led to new behaviors and blah, blah, blah, blah.

Wow, that's exhausting just to type, let alone read, isn't it?

Can you feel my drive to explain and link? Where's my advanced "avatar-like" capacity to appreciate the unpredictable emergence in Life, not to mention surrender to mystery and not knowing? (That annoying niyama of Ishvara Pranidhana.) If only I would just give you a story of precisely why all this pain led to my present day experience, then you too could feel safe and share such exacting stories with your students, repeating the samskara of our collective past due to our clamor to reach a safe place or *home* à la Rohr. Given what we have explored together thus far, that certainty tale is no longer a very satisfying story though either, is it? Can we be OK in the paradox of not really knowing *and* being confident we also understand now? *Docta ignorantia* embodied? That paradox is related to that oft-quoted bit about journeying only to arrive where we started. So here I sit right now (albeit comfortably now) in the exact same recognition of mystery I was in the cabin, but full of joy in my realization that I *am* creativity. I hope you can take at least some small part of that joy as we move into the fun of creativity.

Bridging from Pain to Creativity

Eros drives the universe. One galaxy devours another, supernovas birth new galaxies, the passion of hormones in adolescence, the search of the fruit fly in the kitchen, and the tender last caress of the life mate of 60 years as the other surrenders their final exhale. Only humans could make such an innate quality of life such as Eros complicated. Our sensual, sensing, sense-making nature has been creating stories about creation as far back as we can see. I have written a graduate textbook on the topic and mercifully refer you to it if you are seeking that depth of inquiry (Taylor 2015b). In this chapter we will briefly describe our relationship with what creativity is and isn't, then how it relates to yoga and pain, the ongoing science into creativity, how we can prime ourselves to optimally express it in teaching and business, and, finally, the implications for creating our best futures.

Our operating premise has been that yoga is not a thing, but a "how" of relationships. Yoga therefore is evolving as an ongoing creation or expansion of consciousness and awareness. Creativity and destruction rest in a tension of polarity common within wisdom paradoxes. As we explore creativity's relationship with pain and suffering, bear in mind the first step to creativity is destruction. Rohr (2013) asserts that, until someone walks with the personal existential issue of despair, they won't uncover the wisdom on the other side of that despair. Destruction occurs when we finally allow the crash and crush of our inaccurate and superficial images. Then we discover the wisdom beyond that of what only *seems* like death before the destruction. That death is an imaginary loss of an imaginary self, which is going to pass anyway and informs the klesha of abhinivesha. It is this discovery from our pain and suffering that reveals a creative perception of disharmony in our process of thought and can permit us to come upon the deepest harmony that is open to us. But we get ahead of ourselves. Let's first destroy your understanding of what creativity is. You know the drill by now: Introduce complex topic, destroy the "clods," prepare to harvest the bounty because of our new understanding.

What Creativity Is and Is Not

Our understanding of creativity has been shaped by our cultures, our beliefs in what and who we are, and our professional education's biases about how we deliver yoga services and why. I promised a new definition of creativity after we destroyed your present definition. Well, let's mix things up and let me offer this one as a replacement. Afterwards we will break up what was probably part of your old definition just to be creative.

As yoga professionals, consider this one and change it as you wish as you read further and we unpack it a bit:

> Creativity in yoga is our (yours and the student's) participation more fully in practices that facilitate the emergence of a renewed flourishing of our being at home in our circumstances.

Creativity takes us back to our first biology class where we discovered the characteristics of living things. The ability to respond and adapt to our environment is one of those basic qualities that separate us from non-living things. Creativity is also a current hot topic in the popular media and business press. By the number of books and blogs on creativity one would think the topic is something that is well studied and understood. Unfortunately neither is correct.

The short version of the story is that our current understanding of creativity has been shaped by three powerful forces:

1. Cultural biases and limitations: Ever wonder why the creatives are almost entirely men, individuals, and hailed as geniuses?

2. The methodologies for understanding employed by the cultures: That means the mechanistic worldview we thoroughly explored in the wisdom chapter and a failure to employ complex thinking and emergence within living systems.

3. The epistemological (how we come to know reality) factors that ground those methodologies: Our hubristic quest for certainty,

trying to describe the one, "real" way reality is rather than assuming the humility of wisdom.

Those biases leave us with a thin current accepted general definition of creativity that reads something like "to bring something new and adaptive into the world." Rather bland and leaves open many questions and misconceptions, especially when applied to working with complexity inside wisdom traditions. We need a deeper exploration for our work here. Questions such as, "What is characteristic of the results of creative action, for example the pain theory, the surgical technique, the yoga intervention, the student adapting to a chronic pain condition, and so forth?" David Bohm wrote that we should distinguish between an occasional act of penetrating insight and the discovery of something new that is really creative. In the latter, he said that there will be a perception of a new basic order (of relationship) that is potentially significant in a broad and rich field. This new order in our work should lead eventually to the creation of "new structures having the qualities of harmony and totality, and therefore the feeling of beauty" (cited in Nichol 2006, p.8). Those are a rich bunch of yoga-like words, no? Let's harrow our clods some more to raise our awareness about our assumptions and be grounded in the deeper wisdom of Bohm's and our definition.

Try saying these out loud to yourself, noting which ones are easy and which ones don't come out so smooth. The clunky ones are your clods.

Creativity is:

- an emergent process, not a skill or talent

- a way each of us can operate, not limited to a few

- something that rests on traditional rigorous disciplines, not an abandonment of tradition

- embedded in our many environments and dependent on interaction with others, not expressed in isolation

- a process that emerges from the practice of other behaviors you practice, not a thing you do

- something the brain participates in and is changed in the process, but not a pattern of brain activity

- fundamental to evidence-based healthcare

- not easy or simple, but worth the risk and effort compared to the boredom of the rote and safe

- something we do "with," not to, students when we do a best practice of yoga

- stifled by institutions and systems processes as threatening despite lip-service to the contrary

- useful and practical

- knowing enough, with some expertise, but also cultivating an outsider mindset to avoid constraining thinking and perspective

- not limited to a breed, expert or personality type

- a process of incubation, integration, and implementation rather than a mere Eureka moment

- novelty that comes from the combination or application of other knowledge, and is neither wholly original nor without context

- driven by intrinsic motivation and often aligned with intrinsic desires

- composed of various stages, but not some fixed, linear creative method (from creative problem solving to design thinking)

- supported by constraints and can generate conflict, so tranquility is not a prerequisite

- in line with ethics and should add to the flourishing of life, not be value free

- recognized in one another (student and professional), not what we give or sell

- collaborative, mutual learning within many contexts (transcontextual).

Did any of the descriptions trip you up at all? Any surprises? Every time I rewrite or revisit this list, I discover some new perspective or facet of creativity. Next let's try on a few more ways of saying what creativity is for our many audiences.

Creativity has been defined as an emergent process, arising out of the interactions of a given system and therefore unpredictable (Montuori 2011). We can also paraphrase Halifax (2012) by noting how easily creativity mirrors her dynamic systems definition of compassion:

> Compassion [Creativity] is not a discrete feature but an emergent and contingent process that is at its base enactive. Compassion [Creativity] is best primed through the cultivation of various non-compassion [non-creativity] factors. This article endeavors to identify the interdependent components of compassion [creativity].

In short, both compassion and creativity are composed of enactive (how we bring forth meaning via intimate interactions with our environment), engaged, emergent processes that arise out of the interaction of a number of non-compassion and non-creative processes. What I find especially fascinating is that there are many shared processes between our value of compassion as it relates to wisdom within our vocation and our present quest for understanding creativity. Aren't these threads back through our earlier chapters satisfying to discover? Here are a few more threads.

Creativity can be considered a process that is grounded in interrelationality and incomplete in isolation. It is mutual, reciprocal (affected by relational interaction), and asymmetrical, meaning it does not represent some equilibrium between participants, but has variable degrees of contribution (Montuori 2011). You and your student(s) are not creative without the relationship between all of you, and your mutual interactions from all your systems of experience, which, while initiated and supported by you, only occurs because of "smaller" concurrence and participation by everyone. Together while teaching we foster an aspect of cultivation and nurturing much like planting a seed. Initially the asymmetry may appear to be one direction (the teacher as one who plants and tends). But then, in the harvest, the other party's contribution may emerge in wholly unexpected and surprising ways much like a plant nourishing others or a sapling growing into a tree, offering a lifetime of aesthetic pleasure and resources. We cannot say how the creations of life challenges, to include my Minnesota experience, will create future scenarios. We also don't know how our understanding of creativity in the future will change as well.

The idea of creativity undergoing ongoing evolution and creation leaves a "firm" definition of creativity appropriately uncertain and shifting. Montuori (2017) is interested in how we have created our understanding of creativity because:

> our understanding of creativity is, after all, also a creation. Creativity is evolving, meaning at least that human beings construct an understanding of what this thing or process is that they call creativity, and that this understanding changes over time. We are now at an important turning point where our understanding of creativity is undergoing a considerable transformation. (pp.147–156)

He wisely cautions that, during times of transformation, it is important to review where we've been to better sense where we might be going, and to also "avoid the embarrassing and potentially dangerous possibility of thinking we're changing when in fact we're just doing the same old thing, and making the same old mistakes" (2017, p.147). I echo his sentiment, hence the breadth and depth of this coverage of creativity in this chapter. It is worth our effort to spend some time here to avoid the same old mistakes of *unskillful benevolent responses*.

The Creativity to Yoga Connections

It is often said that yoga is union or yoking. We now have modern names to add to our definition. Transcontextual, mutual learning, symmathesy, and complexity are just a few as we cultivate eco-literacy: understanding the interdependencies. Now there is even a paradigm of the *creative universe*. Creativity in that view is no longer an extraordinary phenomenon isolated in a few gifted individuals. Rather, creativity has a central role, larger than the individual, or *transpersonal* in the sense that creativity is connected with the very nature of our world. The space, the rocks, the stars, thoughts, you name it. Can you see why we had to do all the fieldwork of the previous chapters? This transformation requires us to think and sense very differently. The early chapters have brought us to an appreciation of the way our yoga understanding yields creativity from modern pain science, wisdom practices, and our yoga therapy.

Capra and Luisi (2016) illustrated how the best of science now weaves life and creativity in a relationship that fits our operating yoga definition. If we zoom into the level of the cell (I promised no quantum stuff, this is as far in as we're going), life itself is understood as an emergent property. Realize that none of the basic constituents of a living cell: nucleic acids, proteins, lipids, polysaccharides, and so on, are alive by themselves. However, when they all come together (yoke?) in a particular space/time situation, life, the ultimate emergent property, arises. In our systems language, the spontaneous emergence of order at critical points of instability is one of the most important concepts of the new understanding of life. The same principle of emergence we described about pain is also one of the hallmarks of life itself. Incredible. Creativity has been recognized as the dynamic origin of development, learning, and evolution. In other words, creativity, as the generation of new forms, is a key property of all living systems. Recall CDSR, Complex:Distributed:Self-organizing:Representational. This same emergence is an integral part of the dynamics of open systems, and open systems develop and evolve. Life constantly reaches out into novelty and, according to Gaia theory, life creates the conditions for its own existence (Capra and Luisi 2016). We do not live in a deterministic world of Newtonian billiard ball relationships, where there is no history and no creativity and one thing just directly causes the next thing predictably. Our living world of self-organizing and emergent structures is where history and relationships play an important role. The future is uncertain and this uncertainty as we are appreciating is at the heart of creativity. Emergence results not from magic, but as the creation of novelty, and this novelty is often qualitatively different from the circumstances out of which it emerged. Now that is a positive message of possibility for ourselves and those we serve.

These deep science (*sciencia* = knowing) complements our embodied experience in yoga practice of also being and becoming, all three (knowing, being, and becoming) fundamental to all of life and our humanity. These changes in identity beg tough questions. What if we take seriously this idea that we are part of an ongoing creative process, one that began with the creation of the universe? What if the universe is a *creatio continua*, and we, *creatures* that we are, are both created *and* creating in this ongoing creation? As we described, our very understanding of the universe, and of our condition in the universe, is itself a creation. What if our "cosmological motive," the way we make sense of the world and choose to live in the world, is also, and perhaps our greatest, creation? These are just rhetorical questions. They are the foundation for personal ethical review as part of our yamas and niyamas practices. This is the "stuff" of our psychospiritual practice that yields insights and understading to create skillful, benevolent responsiveness. A review of the cosmological story in the Bhagavad Gita ought to shake us to our core in the way it describes what cosmologists describe as the birth of our universe. How did they know?

One way I tell this story of creativity is to use the limited, but familiar, analogy of how our thinking needs to change is somewhat like software updates. Akin to a new operating system update on your computer or phone. It isn't so much that version 1.0 of creativity was wrong, but it was very limited in function, just like that old computer system. As we roll out and create a 2.0 version of creativity, there are many new features to discover, but along the way probably more than a few glitches or awkward learning moments as well. That's going to be fine, as your practices to prime for creativity will also be your built-in and responsive tech support system. The glitches are expected and we know the search for better solutions is the process, not the problem. It is expected we will still creep back from time to time wanting to just know how to do it or how to tell our students do it. Luckily that tendency, by its integral nature, creates its own set of somatic, embodied stress responses that can cue us to reassess our thinking and our actions. The word "radical" describes this change in systems, deriving from the word root. Adopting this new creative operating system is a radical departure from our former understanding. We are back to destruction as it will uproot or disturb nearly all the old roots for us and our students. Therefore. it is important we realize that the adoption of the new software system will be both exhilarating and terrifying at once.

The software tale is simplistic, but one most people can relate to. Our tales interweave in our sense of journey and our stories of the journey, such as the tale of chronic pain. The software story is language we can use and speak to help others understand the value of story and authoring better stories. Montuori (2017) reported that Italian philosophers Gianluca Bocchi and Mauro Ceruti (2002) have explored the many human origin stories, and argue that we live in a *Narrative Universe*, with interweaving stories and multiple narratives. As yoga professionals, we know that the many ways a student describes their world and themselves, in turn shape them. "We create knowledge that in turns creates us, our ways of thinking and acting and feeling" (Montuori 2017, p.152).

One big story told in conventional healthcare for the better part of the last half century is that of evidence-based medicine (EBM). Again, there's an entire chapter in my textbook if this something you can't get enough of here (Taylor 2015b). For our purposes, realize that this is just another story and it creates structures and processes that at times have been co-opted to block or resist creativity. In its original telling, patient circumstance/context and values were primary, followed by and balanced with the provider's clinical mastery and experience, and then whatever literature existed to inform care options. The "evidence" was meant to mean all three, in their order of priority. In the natural evolution of power dynamics and systems dysfunction, too frequently the order has been inverted and often equated to just the last component of "if there's no high-level research dictating practice, it isn't EBM." This is slowly starting to erode back to a healthier balance, but just beware certain audiences might not be receptive to creativity with the same enthusiasm we are sharing in this book. Better to stick with the story that you are using a "BPS approach informed by neuroscience and basic science" for now. I realize it might be tempting to share how ishvara pranidhana comes forward in what Merton called the faith in the myth of the authority of science. He noted that the uncertainty principle was likened to:

> As God in the highest eludes the grasp of concepts, being pure Act, so the ultimate constitution of matter cannot be reduced to conceptual terms. There is, logically speaking nothing there that we can objectively know… This seems to me to be the end of conventional nineteenth century materialism. (cited in Fox 2016, pp.53–54)

A monk reveals a niyama via physics. Now that's creative. But resist the temptation to lead this response.

A similar caution about matching story to audience is highlighted by O'Donohue. He observed that life must be a creative act because he'd met humans looking for all kinds of things. He stated though that he never met a human who responded to his question "What are you looking for on this day?" with "I'm looking for yesterday. Where did yesterday go to?" In telling this story, he was suggesting how important it is to help us and our students stay grounded in the present. Even though we are comfortable with the fact that yesterday goes into nothingness, we so often spend much of our lives there. And if not in the yesterday, equally ineffectively, we dwell in the future where we have no idea what will land on the "shoreline of morning tomorrow" (O'Donohue 2017). While we do naturally move through these places, as we are always actively involved in receiving and shaping our lives, where we find creativity unfolding is in the present. The setting of our stories matters, and staying aware of "Long, long ago" or "Someday I'll" are important cues to listen for from both our stories and the students that indicate not being in the present.

So, is there really a science of creativity? There is not "a" single science, but, not too surprisingly, many parts that are trying to "know"/ *sciencia*. Let's look at some more fascinating linking of the diverse views and differentiate those views to break up clods of rigidity.

What Is Creativity Science?

Just as the word yoga carries many preconceptions/misconceptions, so too does creativity. The images range from a disheveled artist's gallery, the play areas at Google, the mad professor's laboratory, to the fun of a desert transformed for Burning Man. For you to try to convince a conservative student or buttoned-down neurologist that yoga therapy is a creative response for chronic pain, well, that just might not go well given those stereotypes. In this section I will share some talking points so you can create the proper, "serious" context of creativity being safe and effective.

The first point is that creativity is not a free for all and that every or anything is creative. As we defined above and described EBM, a creative response to chronic pain should have the outcome of flourishing (toward health and wellbeing) as well as improved quality of life (practical, at home). Couple those outcomes with the principle of emergence as the student being part of complex living systems science (they'll nod, not necessarily understanding, but respecting what sounds serious and therefore correct).

Another way to put creativity in context is to say that more and more people are starting to inquire into the question of what creativity is. Our serving someone with a complex, chronic health challenge is a bit like improvisational acting. The complexity means there is no script to follow precisely and the surprises improv are those layers that continue to unfold in response to care and time. This idea of improvisation tests even the best of us with a tension between our professional skills and the improvisation needed to be *skillfully benevolent in our responsiveness, or wise.* (Isn't it handy to have a definition of wisdom?) Who's going to argue, "I don't want to be wise, I just want to be right"? If we bridge these ideas to the fact that there has been a growing body of sciences addressing creativity the past 30 years or more, the idea of creativity grows not only safer, but necessary.

The dominant scientific inquiry into creativity comes from the silos of disciplines with a primarily North American perspective that is based on:

1. The self as the fundamental unit of creativity. (We've already dissected that one.)

2. A limited consideration of the effects of community, tradition, and shared meaning upon the self. (Re-read the wisdom chapter to deconstruct that one.)

3. A bias away from sociological and philosophical principles in discussions. (How wise is it to not include central, existential issues?)

4. A self-concept that prevents an understanding of the many cross-cultural variations in self-concepts. (Which single self are we considering?)

5. Despite a cultural emphasis on freedom of choice and autonomy, there is an unawareness of the subtle but pervasive pressures to conform to be like everyone else at work, at school, and at conferences with colleagues. (These pressures are becoming acutely more powerful by the week it seems.) (Taylor 2015b)

Combine those superficial and inaccurate assumptions together, and then limit the context to a single department or department within a department of study and you can sense the quality of the outcome. Montuori and Purser (1997) used psychology as an example, and offered this partial list of the silos of inquiry that now exist and can inquire into creativity, but not necessarily communicating or utilizing the other sections' insights:

1. psychology alone considers:

   - psychometrics

   - psychohistory

   - social constructionism

   - cognitive psychology

   - systems theory

   - phenomenology

2. anthropological perspectives

3. organizational creativity

4. sociological inquiry into creativity

5. historical examinations of creativity.

This glimpse allows us to appreciate the fracturing of what we consider creativity science and how we end up with so many silly "pop" creativity books and courses such as "Five Easy Ways to Be Creative." Fortunately, there are a growing number of people exploring how we move beyond this piecemeal approach.

The way we need to build this creativity science is a form of what is known as constructivism (build and rebuild as we go). Contrast that with realism (breaking down into enough different parts to describe the one, single, only real way reality exists). This newer approach of constructivism acknowledges, with humility, that every perspective is limited and, therefore, fallible (how many times have you read that already?). Subsequently, our responsibility (and privilege) is to construct multiple ways of describing a reality that is dependent on who is doing the inquiring and with what tools are they looking. This multiplicity of descriptions generates, for someone operating in the realism view, a very frustrating plurality of reality. Keeping this science stuff simple, just appreciate that the structures of our science and education systems have left us with a pile of unlinked differentiated parts of creativity for now.

The systems science discussed in Chapter 3 yields areas we can begin to investigate in terms of creativity when working in a therapeutic relationship. Using Siegel's (2017) language of our science culture, we can ask: Where can novelty emerge that is rooted in compassion/benevolent responsiveness? He describes the system of energy and information flow within and between us in a therapeutic setting as having three characteristics:

1. The flow is open to influences from outside of itself (those many transcontextual symmathesies).

2. The flow is capable of being chaotic, meaning, roughly, it can become random in its unfolding (no orderly development process here).

3. In flow's non-linear emergence, there is the possibility that small inputs lead to large, not easily predictable results.

That's bad science news for those of us wanting that tidy recipe book for eliminating pain. The process is bound to be open, chaos-capable, and non-linear. Siegel acknowledges that, when people hear the term complex, they can become nervous, especially those well-pedigreed in some isolated discipline. Everyone understandably wants more simplicity in their lives. Perhaps we can reassure them that being complicated is not the same as complexity. Complexity is elegantly simple in many ways, as we will soon discover.

By simple I don't mean easy, no effort involved. I refer more to elegance and fitting well. Another word for this idea is harmony. We've observed how self-organization moves a system, naturally, without a programmer or procedure manual, toward maximizing complexity. This natural push toward maximizing complexity is actually quite simple, rather than being complicated, as it is created when we differentiate and link elements of the system. I suspect we have all had that experience when a session just flows and both you and your student are a bit surprised, but relieved at the simplicity involved. That's what I mean by harmony. Siegel uses a choir analogy where members differentiate their individual voices but link at harmonic intervals, a form of self-organization that can provide a deep and powerful sense of vitality. This is a natural self-organizational movement toward harmony and is often a component of creativity that we observe working with our own or others' suffering and pain (Siegel 2017).

How will we balance simplicity and harmony, with dominant cultural drive for "the more information and data is better to get closer to having the entire representational map of reality"? To make a binary choice of either this or that violates our yoga and wisdom. Both/and of course is the answer. A good first step is if we filter this increasing volume of data with the recollection that the knowledge (how we organize information) that we are constructing is within contexts and dependent on the inquirer (us, and with no more illusion of objectivity). We also have a responsibility to determine what is "worth" knowing given we are constructing our reality. This question brings us to the concept of axiology, the branch of philosophy that deals with values, or, put simply, what is worth knowing? Axiology is a new term to most yoga professionals as it addresses the very subjective practice of acknowledging that what we choose to inquire about regarding reality always involves us as the inquirers. This is in direct opposition to the old realist's quest for a remote, objective, unbiased inquirer. The recent awareness of how media, technology, and our choices drastically bias our understanding of the *news* has at least brought this need to a broader awareness. There are a number of practices ahead to accentuate and clarify our need to decide what is worthy of our time and what will prime deep and accurate insight. We now realize that answering what is worthy of our time based on the science of creativity insists it is us who must decide. More response-ability. For us and our students.

Kauffman (2016) counsels not to let "science" overwhelm us. Inform us, yes. But in balance, he states that our humanity vastly outstrips science, and that it is our humanity and our potential transformation within our civilization that can unleash and serve humanity as we, and those we serve, ever "become" in our unending novelty if we accept that "becoming" as our foremost purpose. Certainly, modern science is superb, he contends, but presently modern science dominates us beyond what we need. Both/and again. He points to what happened when the Renaissance emerged as a new, unprestatable/predictable view of our humanity that ultimately led to modernity via Newton *et al.* We literally describe it as the movement from the Dark Ages to Enlightenment. That wasn't a one-time-only phenomenon, but an example of a harmonious, elegant advancement in complexity that emerged.

Today we are tucked between scientism that plagues us and blinds us and the fact deniers. Another Dark Age of our own. The scientism has made our world devoid of mystery and full of hubris. Kauffman (2016) described how, as a people, we have become disenchanted and many move in a meaningless universe, unable to even consider the *central existential issues* and their choices that should give our lives their meanings. Sounds as though we need creative wisdom. Know any profession that teaches to foster those capacities for both creativity and wisdom? That leads us to our next section.

Who Is Creative?

Remember in the first chapter on yoga we noted the conspicuous absence of half of humanity in understanding what yoga might be and its His-story? Any guesses who has also been left out of the history of creativity and who is considered creative? Montuori (2017) reported the major gaps in gender representation and groups of non-European origin in the history of creativity. So while it might seem obvious today to declare that everyone is creative, such a statement in historical and contextual fact is a radical notion, and still not evident in today's societal structures. The absence of women, people of color, and the imbalanced representation in world organizations demonstrates that deep societal denial of the creative potential of many groups continues. Imagine the polling results in the USA of Arabic, African, Asian, or Indigenous people's contributions to creativity? Sad, but descriptive.

The easy part then is to declare that creativity is a quality of the known universe, not limited to species, or even not only the animate, but also the inanimate. Therefore, we aren't so much creative, as we are creativity itself. Our vocation than becomes transforming society to deeply and accurately reflect that insight into the existential question of what are we. We will begin unpacking that idea a bit more and then look at a few implications for our yoga profession prior to describing practices that prime us to fully be what we are.

As complex beings and considering the prior chapters' description of symmathesies, mutual learning, and emergence, we understand every moment of our life is an invitation to creativity, even in the most ordinary moments. Those ideas have revealed characteristic of complexity that mirrors the yoga concepts of unity in diversity *and* diversity within a unity. Wisdom and yoga view the fabric of life as composed of many threads where one new thread influences the entire fabric. If people seize their ordinary creative power, then extraordinary changes can take place. Our ordinary creativity has tremendous implications when we begin to explore the decades' and centuries' old power dynamics around creativity at the close of this chapter. First, what about our old image of creativity as "special" and reserved for the few?

Montuori shared Maslow's useful distinction between special talent (ST) and self-actualizing (SA) creativity (2017, p.150), special talent being creativity such as that of a musical prodigy or mathematically adept child. Maslow wanted to distinguish this group of people who have a special talent in one specific area from another group that doesn't necessarily have one overriding talent, but for whom creativity is more distributed. The self-actualizing seem to have creativity as a function of their whole life, rather than just one specific talent. The self-actualizers see all of life as an opportunity to be creative. Montuori went on to write that for them creativity is a given, not an exception. They don't summon creativity on certain occasions of need. Rather, they "are" creativity. Their bigger challenge is "channeling that creativity in a way that is good for the particular task" (p.150). Maslow used the term self-actualizing to refer to people who are psychologically healthy and integrated. Sounds like the goal of a yoga practitioner, doesn't it? What other traits do people who are behaving creatively share?

Frank Barron (1990) in his seminal creativity research described traits creative individuals tend to exhibit:

- an independence of judgment rather than conformity

- a tolerance for ambiguity rather than a need for certainty

- a preference for complex thinking rather than polarized, simplistic oppositional thinking

- androgynous behaviors with clarity on gender attributes and roles rather than a masculine preference

- a preference for complexity of outlook and a tolerance for asymmetry rather than symmetric, constrained possibilities.

How do these traits match up with those in positions of power and influence today? By extrapolation, do they reflect the traits of organizations and nation-states around the world? Why might this be the case?

Bohm wrote about the tendency for the pain that arises from the conflict in the mind as it tends to try to escape awareness rather than accurately respond to what is happening. We can apply this both individually and collectively, I suspect. He brilliantly stated that as the mind does this, it does so by initiating a state of confusion. Might he be describing vrittis here? He went on to describe how, "when the mind is trying to escape the awareness of conflict, there is a very different kind of self-sustaining confusion, in which one's deep intention is really to avoid perceiving the fact, rather than to sort it out and make it clear" (cited in Nichol 2006, p.27). Ouch. That's certainly me in the reflection and much of the dynamics is politics and government today.

He offers some hope when he writes that it seems that we each in our own way have to discover what it means to be original and creative. His encouragement continues, stating that "generally speaking, the childlike quality of fresh, wholehearted interest is not entirely dead in any of us. It comes in a small burst, and then it gets lost in confusion as all the old special interests, fears, desires, aims, securities, pleasures, and pains come up from the past" (p.27). What a treat to have a nuclear physicist explain samskaras in such simple language. He tackles vrittis again, pointing out that this repeated process/rut creates an order all its own. The rut is "a reflexive state of dullness in which the natural agility of the mind is replaced with torpor on the one hand, mechanical and meaningless fantasies on the other" (p.27). Regrettably, we can observe that this has come to be considered a normal state of mind, and has spread and is spreading throughout our modern culture. His prescription was that we need to give patient, sustained attention to the activity of confusion, rather than attempting to promote creativity directly. For Bohm, and us, as we will see momentarily, giving *simple attention*, a "finer, faster process" than confusion, is itself the primary creative act.

A final consideration is the implication of what Montuori calls reproductive education versus creative inquiry. Is there something in the way we are training yoga professionals that is unwittingly blocking our creativity? Each profession tends to teach from what Montuori (2017) defines as "reproductive" education as the dominant pedagogy. In reproductive education, students are instructed in what is known, what is to be done, and how it is to be done. Students then "pass" if they can reproduce that knowledge as instructed and perform the behaviors of treatment as delineated in yoga educational setting. There is generally not room or credit given for innovation, deviation, or adaptation. Creative inquiry does not exclude this important reproduction of the foundations and traditions. But it also doesn't stop there or declare heretical any deviation from tradition. There is a very real tension between creativity and what I describe as the "fundamentalism" of tradition in yoga. Has that ever been your experience? Have you observed others in that type of environment? This taps into what Montuori (2017) calls the polarities of relationship between innovation and tradition, the individual and society, freedom and authoritarianism, process and essence, and more broadly the central existential issues exploring what we are made of, to include the central metaphor for what life, the Universe, and everything is all about. Creative inquiry in contrast invites us, after gaining the foundations, to a robust exploration, questioning assumptions, enmeshed in mutual learning in a transcontextual manner. Have we arrived back at the wisdom chapter, or are we now just ready to build on it as it weaves through yoga, pain, and creativity?

Priming Skills for Creativity

The world has trained most of us to deny that we are creative. That's where I was in Minnesota, looking outside myself for solutions, and I suspect many of you have been there too. How do we overcome the fixed cultural thought "I am not creative?" There are many factors to address, but a key lies in what David Kelley, co-author of *Creative Confidence:*

Unleashing the Creative Potential within Us (2013) calls creative confidence, a self-concept that claims creativity as a natural-born human ability in all of us. This section is about cultivating and nurturing a kind of fearless confidence we can take from knowing that the capacity for creativity is already not only in us, but is us.

Because we are creativity, there isn't some "thing" we add to create our essence. Instead we use words like prime, nurture, or foster. Gardening metaphors work well: to cultivate, tend, or fertilize. I am partial to Halifax's "priming" as she used that word to break up the notion we can train compassion, another complex emergent human capacity. As we revisit her domain practices for priming, note any tendency of yourself to draft an engineering systems model, and when you do, soften and see if you can allow a messier, multidimensional smear of relationship of mutual learning to unfold. Straight lines of connection and circles are far too clean. We are more like the little old lady's wild, burgeoning overgrown garden at the end of the lane than a tidy British manicured garden. Sunshine, rain, and time allow what is already primed to burst into being.

Range of Imagination

Before going further, it is worthwhile to contemplate the quality with which we hold onto our models of reality as well. How do you "see" this model of priming domains? The panca maya kosha or chakra models? The scientific method of realism? Are you back to clean, crisp engineering diagrams? I like to call this "looking" our "range of imagination" exercise. Bohm offered a great image for softening and smudging our use of models and theories. He noted that the most creative and original aspect of scientific work is the development of theories, especially those that feel to be universally relevant. Why this feeling arises, he speculated, could be that "the word "theory" derives from the Greek 'theoria,' which has the same root as 'theater,' in a verb meaning 'to view' or 'to make a spectacle'" (cited in Nichol 2006, p.53). We can soften to hold our models and theories as primarily the ways we have of looking at the world through our changeable, unique lens of the moment, remembering the unfolding play is just one form of insight (and not a form of knowledge of the exact, one way that the world *is*). Just as our experience of theater is dependent on who we are that day as to whether it moves us or bores us, so too we say that models are ways of looking which are neither true nor false, but rather clear and fruitful in certain circumstances, and unclear and unfruitful when extended beyond these those situations. So, as with all art, can we hold this model as a work that will unfold across time and change as we change? We will *theoria*/see.

Halifax's Adapted Model

This model with the three axes was introduced last chapter in our discussion of pain. The three axes create a *skeleton* that can hold the continual shifting reality of the complex being. Together they contain the infrastructure for describing the ubiquitous yoga marketing description of body–mind–spirit. The dynamism of the axes generates cascading levels of insight and possibility as we play with the recurring, continuous cycles of relationship discovery. Prior to that play, let's briefly revisit each domain available in Halifax (2012).

The attentional/affective axis is the channeling of energy and information flow by how and to what we attend. We have seen this "exercise" leads to activation of neuronal firing and contributes to us becoming attuned to our and the other's affective state. Never in isolation, now we begin to jump between the bones of the axes. Attentional clarity and balance through mindful embodied practices (the E/E axis) results in decreased susceptibility to the effects of emotionally arousing events and task performance (Ortner, Kilner and Zelazo 2007). This embodied attention appears to prime our brain circuits that associate with empathy/affective attunement. Practices from the E/E axis at the same time raise both our inner reality awareness (physical, emotional, and cognitive) and awareness of the external reality with which we are engaged. This balance is dependent, of course, on our awareness of the somatic expressions of emotions that offer insight (I/I axis) which then through our intention to practice compassionately/wisely redirects us to our or the other's affect, and so on, and so on. Can you glimpse the theatrical magic of this illustration and how in a small way the cycles move across the stage in interaction? Mutual learning/growing and flowering. Bravo.

In describing the Intentional/Insight axis, Halifax (2012) asks what processes beyond the Attentional/Affective (A/A) axis allow us to cultivate compassion and not fall into reactions of "avoidance, abandonment, numbness or moral outrage" that would inhibit our rehabilitation care? She proposes that our focused attention and ability to guide our mind with the intention to be compassionate generates insights about the suffering, the suffering's origins, and how to transform suffering in a creative emergence. The double Is of intention and insight refer to our cognitive dimension of experience and, as we've seen, interact in conjunction with the other axes. Reciprocally our intention and insight also prime our attention and affective balance. Again, our complex being reveals that this weave of attentional, affective, cognitive, and somatic domains are interlaced and intimately further associated with our social, cultural, and environmental fabric (Taylor 2015b). Our ability to appreciate a broader stage of the full nature of the suffering (societal, students', and ours) allows for the emergence of novel and effective insight, as well as action not otherwise available in our teaching.

As yoga professionals, the domains of the somatic or physical Embodiment/Engagement axis may be the most familiar, but not what we may have considered to be important in regards to our creativity. We have reviewed the emerging science of how attention, practice, and behavior alter both the function and structure of our very anatomy and physiology via neuroplasticity, epigenetic function, and the exhibition of altruistic behaviors, including compassion. This experiential E/E axis celebrates these new facts and demands our engagement with these domains to foster the greatest emergence of possibility in our yoga practices. Patanjali urged daily practice, not just thinking about yoga. What we sense, how we move, and why we move are essential to our effectiveness and our creative capacity not just at work, but in every aspect of our lives. Can we continue to dismantle the stage sets of walls of separation between how we sit, breathe, sense, and act? This framework of a model itself transforms in the flow of time, giving us "clear and fruitful" appreciation of the theatrical unfolding of creativity.

Who, Me?

The practice across all the domains of integration is easy to map across the technologies of yoga practice. This includes the ethical practices of the yamas and niyamas we explored in the yoga chapter. Weaving among the domains primes for "identity" integration which is so important when pain and suffering has made the old identity "not fit" artistically anymore. The natural push of their lives as complex systems can be liberated with the right focus of not doing something to them, but instead permitting something to be expressed so that the innate drive toward integration as Siegel's (2017) purpose of mind, could make the present self "fit" in the paradox of beauty holding the full spectrum of life. This new fit of identity (identity as *a central existential life issue*) in Kauffman's (2016) words describing mind, is all about the transformation of the presence of possibility (Who can I be? What can I be?) into the knowns of actuality, defined in the shifting emergence of degrees of certainty in the forever unfoldings of self now. Huh? How about: A safe environment for experiencing all three axes helps students more accurately realize who they are in this moment? So many ways to say the same thing.

Thought as Movements and Asana

Modern postural yoga has inverted the relationship of bodily movement prominent to the psychospiritual development of yoga. Our job now is to bring balance back to an integral understanding of the new yoga. As we are to be able to attend to our thoughts we realize that thoughts are as real a movement as execution of an asana. Thought as movement is that which is actually going on, both inwardly and outwardly, with real effects of significance that interpenetrate and ultimately merge with the whole of who we are and how we live (identity again). Not just little airy thought clouds in isolation. If we fail to give proper attention to these movements as the origin of our and our students' problems, then the very thought that is aimed at solving the problem will be of the same fragmentary and confused nature as that which is producing them, so that what we prescribe will tend to make things worse, rather than better. I am not arguing for a shift to the opposite polarity of psychospiritual inquiry only, rather advocating that we appreciate that these other practices are as equally relevant to easing suffering and pain. Just as with teaching asana movements and alignment while seeking optimization, the alignment/quality of the content of thought may be either "real" or "unreal," with its function nevertheless always real. This function of supporting thought-asana is, first, to give meaning and shape to perception by calling attention to what is regarded as relevant or essential in the context of interest (recall salience and neuroplastic change) and, second, to give rise to awareness of feelings/affect and urges that promote actions/engagement appropriate to the context of the student. How might we "adjust," "prop," and adapt thought to support our students? These thought adjustments would of course have to traverse beyond the skin and skulls of us and our students to our wider environments, circling us back around to organizational yoga. Rest and reflect with the implications of how our practice changes with thoughts as movements and asana. Can you create your own thought-restorative posture so to speak?

We Are Not the Agents

Another caution around our asmitâ-itis. You and I are not the agents of change or creativity. We do not cause or do to the other. That is violence. Our teaching when offered from a wisdom context, merely enables new, typically unpredictable possibles for our students (and us). The agent is their next action in selecting from the new possibles, out which will flow more new actuals as well as more possibles in Kauffman's language (2016). Our teaching then becomes open-ended, creative, beyond predicting rules, and radically emergent. Done well, the practice environment we construct with the student allows for creative perception. We may say that, quite generally, in such creative acts of perception, we and the student first become aware (generally non-verbally) of a new set of relevant differences, and they begin to feel out or otherwise to note a new set of similarities, which do not come merely from past knowledge, but arise in the moment. This movement of thought leads to a new order of self, which then gives rise to a hierarchy of new organization, that constitutes a set of new kinds of understanding and motivations to act in new manners of expression (aka asana). Bohm noted the outcome, or fruit of that practice, is "The whole process tends to form harmonious and unified totalities, felt to be beautiful, as well as capable of moving those who understand them in a profoundly stirring way" (cited in

Nichol 2006, p.20). Said another way by Kauffman (2016), the simplest idea is that mind acausally (enables not causes) selects (a movement), and that movement then converts possibles to actuals. I don't see we teachers as the agents or healers in either description, just the students in their selection. Do you? Good, now let's examine our being agents of change and creativity.

From Idea to Implementation

> "Ideas are a dime a dozen, and the implantation is everything."
>
> (John Bogle, founder of Vanguard Funds, cited in Robbins and Mallouk 2017, p.211)

This section is an entire chapter in my textbook (Taylor 2015b). What do we do with our fount of new ideas and insights as we prime for creativity? What should our students do? The short answer is to pick up David Allen's classic *Getting Things Done* (2002) and Govindarajan and Trimble's *Beyond the Idea* (2013). These two resources have been invaluable to me. They are simple to access, while addressing the complexity of implementation. They all echo Bogle above who shook the financial world and brought great opportunity for the small investor. Allen's getting ideas done is the tough side of Govindarajan and Trimble's two-sided coin of great ideas on one side, and implementation on the other side. What we are talking about here is the *engagement* axis of Halifax. The *skillful action* of the Gita. The *skillful benevolent responsiveness* of wisdom. All done through our embodied enaction in our respective environments.

If we are going to "go" with this symmathesy and mutual learning stuff, we have to accept that I cannot tell you specifically what steps you need to implement your insights. And you cannot do so for your students. To do so is disempowering and a form of Montuori's reproductive education (2017). Create resilience and safety for yourself and the students. Do the practices and *engage* the *insights* with *intention*, *affective* regulation, *attention* and fully *embodied*. To borrow from Rohr (2011), it is as simple as that, and as hard as that. Sorry. Now, what about that business of yours as an area that will require implementation?

Creativity in Business

Another section worthy of its own book. We are always creating our business. The concern is if your business is being created with intention and attention as a form of engaged practice? There is the real possibility that, as you deepen and increase the accuracy of your insights, your present business model will almost certainly no longer be satisfying. I don't mean to imply wisdom progress is to become larger and more profitable. Nothing wrong if it does, but what is essential will be the qualitative shifts you make and that could include scaling back or down. What I want to convey is, as you travel your wisdom arc of development, impermeability will affect your business from your within as well as from without. All of those inner and outer forces of change will come to bear. The death and birth of business cycles. Business is just a specific example of the implementation we just discussed. Kauffman had a nice frame I have borrowed to make this constant cycle of change less serious and threatening. Notice if it might support you too as we ride the process of business development and change.

Earlier we discussed improvisational theater. I, along with Kauffman (2016), believe it is more than just a metaphor for our lives. In improv, the rule is one person must accept the other's line and build on it in a context-appropriate, but unpredictable way. "Yoga can help your back pain," you say. "My mother broke her hip in a yoga class," says the prospective student. You say what? If we can relax into this constant improv rather than being right or making the sale, we discover that each line/exchange does not cause but enables a therapeutically appropriate adjacent set of possible responses. We need to let go, in humble realization that business is just a series of unpredictable sets of possibilities for your next line. Can we listen and wisely respond? If so, as we go around we create a "skit" none of us could have planned, but grounded in wisdom and holding a safe space for their suffering. Together we jointly co-created the skit, not knowing what we would need to do or how we could be of service. I have observed both in my business, and those with whom I have offered consultation, that this more relaxed letting come stance of improv created new business I couldn't have predicted. Played well, who knew you might arrive at, "She will be so relieved I met someone that can safely guide her return to yoga. She was concerned she would never be able to practice. And I have hope for my own back pain relief too!"

Proceed with confidence, humility, and the fun anticipation of improv. Life is full of surprises. We might as well soften into that fact and have fun rather than resisting. So, while I have you at ease, let's check back in with that idea around asmitâ-itis and how stepping up to the full power of our yoga therapy practice might find us onstage with actors we haven't yet ever imagined.

Organizational Yoga Therapy

In the implications of the new yoga chapter I introduced the idea of organizational yoga therapy. If we want to wisely address pain and suffering, we need to effectively dance with the paradox of pain and suffering being both personal and not. It would not be wise to ignore what we do know about ignorance from of all those insights. Plus keep in mind the tendency toward the asmitâ of both the student, and us as yoga professionals, being separate and therefore thinking we are the sole creators/fixers of suffering. You might want to reread that section if it was your first exposure to those ideas.

What becomes clear in looking through the lens of organizational yoga therapy is that the world, society, and human beings are creative processes. As a result, we have created societies, institutions, and relationships that have the implicit, and often explicit, purpose of drastically limiting our creativity. Can you sense the wide and intimate relationship this often unintentional blocking of creativity and resulting suffering represents? Viewing ourselves as a part of a larger cosmic process of creativity and seeing the whole world around us as a creative process involves a process of "re-cognition," an unveiling of the creativity that is always there as part of our heart chakra/hands and voice doing the heart's work. That work on an individual basis is driven by that one unique, unstruck sound we are here to contribute to the creating, creative universe. It also invites us to ask, what are we doing with this innate power of us being creativity? What kinds of institutions, cultures, relationships, are we creating? This entire concept is just emerging as we described. Will we have a hand in this emergence? Here are some new possibles to consider given where we have journeyed in this book so far.

The Future

Now that we have seen the "future" changing nature of yoga therapy, how might new possibles unfold? We can appreciate that the becoming of our biosphere is beyond laws and predictability. This becoming of our future is radically emergent. As a consequence, our answers to *quo vadis* (where are you going?) and how are you going, are very murky when we cannot design but must grow, ever partially unknowing, what we will become (Kauffman 2016). The universe is truly a *status nascendi*, a becoming. This becoming needs to be the center of our new view of ourselves and reality.

This new orientation will need a new story. As we sit with the pain and suffering of existence, realize our guide could be a new origin mythic structure that reflects this new center where we are all fully living and keep becoming vs. a static, wind-up game board. Our responsible, skillful benevolent free will choices are now understood to occur in the context of our capacities, our context, and our purpose. Wisdom grounds our actions and can be explained in terms of reasons, motives, and purposes, including finding unprestatable/unpredictable new purposes. Without such context and capacities, we and our students would have no reasons, purposes, or motives. Those first two limbs are so important.

All of this brings home the tremendous response-ability implied in our creating. Our future reality does not exist until we choose to experiment by asking nature/reality a question, and then mutually learning with nature's answer, which we do by measuring, or our inference. Back and forth in Bateson's symmathesy, we jointly co-create reality. Kauffman describes this as the enigma of our nature. "Reality seems to require us. Reality does not exist separately from us!" (2016, p.175).

If we accept such a premise, then we and our students surely cannot afford to be eco-illiterate. Earlier, in Chapter 3, we equated eco-literacy with health and with what we teach as yoga professionals. Complementing that concept, I discovered that Bohm proposed we need to understand the underlying relationships between art, mathematics, and science ecologically in this new light (Nichol 2006). He noted the origins of these various words indicate a similarity in their original intent: "art" originally meant "to fit"; "science" originally meant "to know"; 'mathematics" originally meant "to know" or "to learn." In Bohm's view, all of these concepts come together in the original meaning of good: "gather," "together," "to join," and, by extension, "fitting together." Bohm arrived then at a working definition of "the good" that was not burdened with moral injunctions, but, rather, described the coherent functioning of the human being (the humanities), and was consistent with the implications of contemporary physics of his day. Isn't the weave he created via these three interrelated factors inspiring? The art/science/mathematics fitting together/good. And, of course, "good" has its roots in "God." How are we going to do likewise as "yoga" teachers?

Can we reveal the unbroken and undivided movement in nature, the inseparability of human experience from that movement, and the wise use of the artistic and the scientific sensibilities to discern the ever-changing meaning of "fitting" and "the good" within that movement? We began with simple movement as asana in our culture. This grander movement that together constitutes the basis for the worldview, Bohm called *artamovement* (Nichol 2006, p.xxiv). Isn't that another beautiful word of depth and richness for describing our becoming world?

Some road signs, or indicators, that our creative process of generating artamovement and less future suffering have been described to guide and encourage us. One such pointer is that we become sensitively aware of how the whole process works, in ourselves and in others. This awareness leads us to to discover that the mind is beginning to come to a more natural state of freedom, in which all our conditioning is seen to be the triviality that it is. What you might notice is that originality and creativity begin to emerge, not as something that is the result of an effort to achieve a planned and formulated goal, but rather as the stabilization of a mind through your priming practices. We are also cautioned that this is the only way in which originality and creativity can possibly arise, since any effort to reach them through some planned series of actions or exercises is a denial of the very nature of what we hope to achieve.

For this reason, originality and creativity can develop only if they are the essential force behind the very first step. This means that it is up to each person to make the first step for themselves. This without following another, or setting up another as the authority for defining what creativity is and for advice on how it is to be "obtained." Unless one starts to discover this for themselves, rather than trying to achieve the apparent security of a well-laid-out pattern of action, they will just be deluding themselves and wasting their efforts. Note how this is reinforced as *empowering* in our yoga therapy definition as well. A subtle, but important, practice of non-harming. My lesson from the cabin too.

Don't be lulled, however, into equating being natural in the expression of our creativity as being easy, for to realize this fact is very difficult indeed. Bohm posts a warning sign that: After all, for thousands of years, we have been led to believe that anything and everything can be obtained if only we have the right techniques and methods (Nichol 2006). As the sages have also noted, what is needed is to be aware of the ease with which the mind slips comfortably back into this age-old mechanistic pattern/samskaras. Bohm acknowledged that certain kinds of things could be achieved through techniques and formulae, but originality and creativity were not among these. The act of seeing this deeply and accurately (and not merely verbally or intellectually) is also the wisdom of action through which originality and creativity can be born (Nichol 2006).

O'Donohue (2017), through his gift with language, made some commentary that is related to Bohm's concept of artamovement. He noted that the Greek root for the word "beauty" is related to the word for "calling," to "*kalon*" and "*kalein*." That origin of the word means that in the presence of beauty, it's not a neutral thing, but it is actually calling you. This hearkens back to our fourth chakra notion of being called. We are constantly being called to be ourselves and called to transfigure what has hardened or got wounded within us as our spiritual practice. It is important we and our students can stay alert to the heart of creativity, as a calling forth all the time, not just occasionally. This is our reality because we are always at a new place, and, if we are aware, then we are also suddenly surprised by where we have been taken to, even in our pain and suffering. Could this pain somehow be what we needed to push against in order to grow? Isn't it sad that we've even commodified growth as an individual as something we can buy and have delivered, versus the mystery of unfolding that life is? I agree with O'Donohue (2017) that even when life delivers something very "negative" or not beautiful, in our judgment, there can be a dialectic there, as he acknowledged that, "the forces are not kind, in terms of beauty, but that actually, those forces could be the impetus and the spur to us to express beauty in our response?" His statement creates a felt sense within me much like a quiet, spectacular sunset. Beauty will be explored further in the practices, but, for now, how do his words create an environment within you?

A final road marker from Fr. Rohr (2017). He reflected that it takes gasping several times in our life to eventually rest in a "bright sadness": "you are sad because you now hold the pain of the larger world, and you wish everyone enjoyed what you now enjoy; but there is brightness because life is somehow, on some levels, still 'very good,'…" He added that Merton said this best, "It does not matter much [now], because no despair of ours can alter the reality of things, or stain the joy of the cosmic dance which is always there… We are [now] invited to forget ourselves on purpose, cast our awful solemnity to the winds and join in the general dance."

Resting in the wisdom of these various markers, I invite you to ask more questions about our becoming, as I did during my research for this book. I discovered, as with everything else we've explored, the list of possibles that become Kauffman's new actuals leading to new possibles in yoga therapy is something we cannot know for certain. What follows here then are some uncertain, but educated speculations from my inquiry of our cosmic dance. A nice summary of my recent observations of how yoga therapy is being delivered in the USA is also available (Taylor and McCall 2017). Jot down any new insights or ideas around what "good" might be and how beauty arises for you as you read through this section. There are practices ahead that will explain how you might then act on these same insights.

The Workplace

We are already witnessing the levels of suffering and pain around the loss of meaningful and living wage employment. The acceleration of change that will continue in our world is all but guaranteed. If jobs aren't lost directly, then the type of work will change and how the person interacts with others will change as well. If we are going to prevent future suffering, how can yoga therapy address this inevitability? We will need to empower students to be able to see a world of creative connection where they can't now see one. Yoga will need to invite exploration into the many ways in which their relationships, from the most intimate to the most commonplace, everyday, work relationships can be an opportunity to connect and create. We now understand that the real life, vocational application of the yamas and niyamas as tools to transform identity around self is more important than another chest-opener series of asanas.

Can you create mutual learning environments to ask if they are seeking to control others, to constrain their self-expression in their work, to have to conform to the picture others have decided they want their work to be, or are they allowing themselves and others to speak, to be who they are and be safe in the work environment? Do they know how to listen in a way that allows their creativity and that of others to flourish in shifting work settings? If they are managers or owners, what embodied skills will they need to make a space for their colleagues to emerge along with then? Do we know the "yoga" of what Nora Bateson (2017) calls how to look, to listen, to encourage, to play, to engage with others in a way that allows our creativities to connect, so that we may create together? Without meaningful, sustainable work, what chance have we of preventing future suffering? Could that be part of the exponential rise of chronic pain in the world today for we group social primates (how biologists refer to human beings)? And for those with chronic pain, is there work for them? The future "yoga" must ask: Do we know how to engage with creation, and let creation engage with us? Can we be strong and flexible in doing so, not just literally?

Our Environment

As eco-literacy educators, who is going to create environments for engaged protection of our larger environmental needs? There are many exciting new ways this is being prototyped and initiated. Our interface with governmental stakeholders and multinational corporations will be a top-down approach, as mentioned in the organizational yoga therapy. What organic, local community-empowered approaches will be needed to affect meaningful change, to include how the next generation grows up in relationship to the planet? There are many robust, empowering action research methods that will take on equal importance to teaching group asana practice in the training curriculum. Every facet of our work needs to spot the asmitâ-itis and respond skillfully with adaptation and change. These research methods are applied community based "yoga" for creating solutions to current suffering. Asana instruction is actually the easier half. Stay tuned.

Wholesale transformation for caring for our planet is needed given the urgency of climate change and pollution taking place. Who will be the change leaders here? Caring for the larger environment is core to our psychospiritual development and practice. The co-creation role we each have is part of this mystery can be called the conspiracy ("co-breathing") with the divine. Rohr rightly asserts conspiracy is still one of the most profound ways to understand what is happening between "God/The Divine" and our soul (Rohr 2011). An engaged, embodied spirituality must always demonstrate a deep "co-operating" between two. No more convenient separate departments of over here is my personal enlightenment quest and over here is my green behavior checklist. I can't wait to see what we create.

Education

This is one of those problems that everyone realizes exists, but is so laden by layers of systems structures and organizational deadwood, very little is changing. Montuori argues that the machine view of the past and the creative "split" we have been exploring still exists inside most of us, and is "certainly still informing our educational institutions, which now have found solace in Ritalin and other drugs when youngsters won't sit still and be a cog in the wheel of the well-oiled machine" (2017, p.149). There are some brilliant exceptions, of course, but what will need to occur to make education anew? And not just for the children, but equally important, for those who are called to educate? Another complex tangle where, right now, most of the time mutual learning, ironically, isn't happening.

Does yoga have anything to offer that would revitalize education in how future generations develop in some way drastically different than the present system? Can we lead the dialog on what education might be? How can it best prepare the students for a future we cannot predict? Might the "problems" of both education and the tidal wave of aging boomers merge to create something that is benevolent and wise? The increments of mindful practices in education being initiated are good first steps, but not if they just allow students and faculty to survive in an ongoing, dysfunctional system. My mind reels with so many ideas of how we could deploy yoga therapy, as I suspect yours does as well. This brings us back to that second side of the innovation coin. Ideas are the easy side. Who will step up to implement and what will we implement?

We need to also remember that we can no more "do to" a system than we ought to "do to" a student. Note how we can pull the threads from the environmental section above to include the politically empowering action research methods I suggested. They are hallmarked for that very reason. You and I don't necessarily have to know the "how." We need only create a space for the process of the larger system to re-cognize what might be done next and then act wisely in a new first experiment. The stakeholders have the solutions, not us.

Siegel offers a great example that I find supportive in letting go of our tendency to need to know what to do next (à la Montuori's "mechanistic still exists inside most of us"). Siegel described how way down at the gene level, during encoded protein building, via the genetic syntax and grammar, there is a process that enables cells to maintain collectively autocatalytic closure (their identity, i.e., the education system) *and* readily explore the enormous explosion of novel proteins and all their potential functionalities (i.e., new education), in the evolution of the biosphere (i.e., our rapidly changing world). So the cells maintain current operations at the same time they are evaluating potential new functions. We need to trust that our grammar and syntax in language as part of the education is just like that in cellular DNA in that it "does not cause, but enables, very complex behaviors to emerge" (Siegel 2017, p.201). What a "conversation" of grammar and syntax this will be within the system charged with teaching grammar and syntax. All I know is, it won't be just your lunchroom or PE asana class anymore making those changes. There is so much that needs to emerge beyond that.

Healthcare

Now here's a system that needs healing. Just apply what I wrote above in the earlier futures sections to all the woes of healthcare and we're just about finished with this section. Seriously. Go back and reread each, substituting these constituents (healthcare consumers and providers). The transcontextuality becomes so apparent, doesn't it? We simply can't tug on one thread without tugging on all the other threads (work, environmental health, education, etc.). And that's good. The weave of complexity remember allows small changes to create large, distant changes that couldn't be predicted ahead of time. We need some of those. My own Minnesota tale being a direct example of a small spark now providing a platform for fanning the fires of change in healthcare on both a national and international level.

I do have a couple of additional perspectives to share beyond the "find and replace" exercise I just suggested. The first is around what might take place in the experience of a therapeutic encounter when done in a yogic manner. Per Siegel (2017), experience is the streaming of energy and information flow, "between and within us" among individuals, and through the body and its brain. He argues that attention is the process that directs the flow of that energy and information and can be generated "in communication between people as well as within people" (2017, p.171). This experience in the therapeutic encounter is about us as yoga professionals as well. Follow along a bit, it is fascinating and ties directly to our domain practices.

He noted that how *attention* is directed to that flow will activate certain neural pathways that create certain interpersonal experiences. In other words, our attentional skills within us make possible attention that drives the activation of neurons in our brain, at a minimum, but more likely an inner attention also drives energy flow throughout our whole body. Our skillful shifting of external attention is a new possible to alter the internal neural firings that shape not only the activity in the brain in the moment, but also "alter the structural connections in the brains of those engaged in the interactions, in the communication, among people…" (p.180). When we recontextualize yoga as skill development where the outcome is that mind can drive energy and information through the body and brain in new ways, even ways that might not happen automatically, those are some exciting new possibles. Such neural activation driven by mental effort with *intentional focus of attention* in specific ways might create many new possibles via different patterns of brain firing than might happen ordinarily. Recollecting our neuroplastics discussions, even though I cautioned regarding overenthusiasm around "neuro," we do have evidence that this mental initiation of brain activity can activate genes, change enzyme levels that repair the ends of chromosomes, and even alter epigenetic regulation of gene expression. Can you glimpse how your mental *intention* and *embodied attention* shape your internal experience (*affective* experience) with your mind, and change your body beyond just building a yoga butt or shoulders? This new construction may also include the various molecular relationships that control neural and bodily function if we continue the relationships and learning that take place. Seigel concludes, using one of the metaphors we earlier described, "You can intentionally shape your mindscape" (2017, p.184). How's that for a healthcare transformational tagline?

The other perspective I wanted to share is wisdom from David Bohm (Nichol 2006). As we sit at the foot of this monstrosity of a mess called healthcare, remember this from his *artamovement* earlier in the chapter. He charged readers that in this art of life we need to be both creative artists and skilled artisans. As we engage, we are always in the act of *fitting* an ever-changing reality, remembering there is no fixed or final goal to be attained. Rather, the moment-to-moment end and the means are both our best *skillful responses* in action to make every aspect (of health) fit. His notion of fitting extends into all of life, to include our limbs called "moral" or "ethical" and that has to do with "the good." Good (God?) as we explored earlier comes from an Anglo-Saxon root (the same as that of "gather" and "together") which means "to join." Ah, there's some yoga/yuj/yoke. These early notions of "the good" imply some kind of "fitting together" in all that humans do, or in being healthy/whole. He shares O'Donohue's love of words, adding that the Latin words *bene*, meaning "good," and *bellus*, meaning 'beauty," are related in origin. Add to O'Donohue's use of beauty earlier, "to fit in every respect," and we could say that such a significance of "the good" is relevant to healthcare becoming healthy. Systems that restrict access, are controlled by profit-seeking institutions with toddler-level consciousness, and encourage passive, disembodied participation à la Sat Bir Khalsa's talk are not healthy. Rather, the good/healthy is that which fits, not only in practical function and in our affective and aesthetic sensibilities, but also that which, by its action/engagement, leads to "an ever-wider and deeper sort of fitting, in every phase of life, both for the individual and for society as a whole" (Nichol 2006, p.106). How can your yoga service lead to better fitting?

Political Power

Matthew Fox (2004b) has been one of the writers that has most influenced my life. I recommend his books on creativity in general, but want to highlight his wisdom from what he calls *creation spirituality*, in describing the relationship between creativity and power. The four paths he shares are embodied and grounded in wisdom traditions, and therefore "yoga." They are:

Via Positiva: The path of wonder and awe.

Via Negativa: This is the path of letting go and letting be in solitude and silence, but also of undergoing grief and sorrow; it's an ongoing act of radical trust in the Divine (ishvara pranidharana).

Via Creativa: This is the path of celebration and creativity, of co-creating with the work of the Holy Spirit.

Via Transformativa: This is the path of compassion and justice; it is the way of the prophet who calls each us into action…to enact in the world in order to help others (p.81). He sums up this section when he wrote "Justice and compassion are not only the test of healthy creativity, they are also the result of healthy creativity" (p.113). This is another way of expanding the yoga expression that the fruits of a proper yoga practice are "sthira and sukha" or "steadiness and calm." Can there be steadiness and calm without justice and compassion in our expanded definition of yoga therapy?

Montuori has written extensively on these power and political relationships if you seek more understanding. For example, he wrote:

But we see also the relationship between creativity and freedom, creating our lives together, rather than the controlling others, or wanting to be controlled by others, where freedom is curtailed, the range of choices reduced, and our existence boxed-in. Creativity is the response and alternative to authoritarianism, to control societies to our own need to control and be controlled. (2017, p.154)

Does this help explain why I campaigned so hard to have "empower" in the yoga therapy definition given our culture today? Our culture shapes our relationships and our self-identity. Siegel wisely summarized,

"What arises from embracing the reality of both this we self and me self is another simple truth: Kindness and compassion, toward the self of the body and the distributed self of our interconnected lives, is the natural way of integration" (2017, p.329). Apolitical yoga instruction is not worthy of our efforts. We must redefine "power yoga" as we and our students assume our power.

Toward the Discovery Chapter

I am so excited about what lies ahead for us as yoga professionals. Sure, there is much to do, but there always has been and will be. As we prepare to move from mostly conceptual exploration into practices, let's zoom out a bit to assume the fun of being creativity. Bohm championed that the health of the body demands we breathe properly, likewise, whether we like it or not, the health of the whole person requires that we be creative. He specified that "the mind is not the sort of thing that can properly act mechanically" (cited in Nichol 2006, p.29). Our vocation then, first for ourselves, then those we serve is to awaken the creative state of mind which is not at all easy. On the contrary, (remember Bohm was arguably one of the smartest people from the twentieth century) "it is one of the most difficult things that could possibly be attempted" (p.29). Well that doesn't sound very fun, does it? Difficult and fun are not opposites. What if by engaging this difficult task:

> A new possible arises à la Kauffman, that catalyzes an evolutionary shift on the order of magnitude of what the swim bladder did for the first fish that came ashore? Seriously, knowing what we know from the past chapters, we hold the power to not cause but enable "a new adjacent possible set of opportunities for the evolution of the biosphere" (Kauffman 2016, p.184).

> Even more powerfully than the worldwide web, which is a subset of the biosphere, "we are poised as a persistent becoming, a persistent status nascendi in a participatory universe that 'is not,' but 'becomes'" (p.184). How thrilling, and fun, to keep forefront in our awareness that just our being *alive* in the world is more important than knowing.

It would be a relief to celebrate that "No one of us can or will do the weaving, nor will it ever end" (p.255).

Siegel wondered if "the mind can rise above our inborn proclivities of the brain, genetically and epigenetically influenced propensities to impair integration, and move us toward a more helpful and healthful integrated way of being in the world" (2017, p.208)?

If we can let "meaning and purpose unfold rather than make them happen" (p.208)? What happens to "difficult" then?

We are modern-day explorers setting out on what I believe are the most fun and exciting adventures in the his/her-story of humankind. Our vessel is neither ship or spaceship, but the lens of integration that is a technology of inclusion and empowerment we have only just begun to understand. Join me in our next great exploration of the fun of discovery.

6

· · ·

The Fun of Discovery

MINNESOTA ADVENTURE

Fun and pain? Sounds a bit kinky, no? How much fun was I having in Minnesota staring at the ceiling all week and making the tortuous trips to the bathroom the first couple days? Not much, of course. Little did I know, though, that two very important things were happening that would later generate a great deal of fun. The first was that the suffering I was experiencing is one of the strongest motivators in humans. It is often said people will repeat their behaviors and only change when the level of suffering has gotten sufficient to exceed the comfort of maintaining the status quo. I was miserable, and I'm just a bit driven to "do well," so deep beneath the surface I had crossed the line of tolerating this persistent, episodic back pain and was now being stoked (pain metaphor pun intended) to make the effort and take the risks to change things in my life to get out of pain. Not at a conscious level yet, but on reflection I can see I was being inspired to change no matter the cost.

The second thing that was happening, or better said, had happened, that would eventually lead to fun, was that my self-image had changed. I'd enjoyed great health and had had no minor, let alone significant, injuries or illnesses in my life up until that time. I was spoiled, quite frankly. And with being spoiled, imagined myself as invincible at least to the point of being able to work as hard and as long as I wanted without limitation. The experience of nearly complete limitation of bed-ridden back pain forced me to see myself otherwise. Such a personal reevaluation or assessment is what informs you and me about two of those key spiritual questions: Who am I? and What am I? In this personal crisis of pain, my image had been transformed. This "me" had limits and was now very motivated to not slam up against those limits again.

The image of old Mr. "Know-it-all" around health and fitness was that I wasn't so fit after all. And for the first time in my life, I was having to be very dependent on others just to get through the day. Not only did that transformation affect my self-understanding, but as you can imagine it radically altered my level of empathy and therefore compassion for those with similar experiences. I hadn't been able to imagine their depth and level of suffering. If only they tried a little harder and did what I told them, they should be getting better. What was their deficit in personality or constitution that was blocking their progress? It surely wasn't my ignorance about the depth and many contributing factors of pain and suffering that was the issue... "I knew stuff about how they ought to be and why they were hurting like they were!" [sic in retrospect]. I didn't know squat.

. . .

The interesting paradox in this level of suffering and self-reassessment has been that it was also the doorway into an unimaginable adventure of discovery and fun. Had my thick veneer of invincibility, and with it a smug sense of clinical self-righteousness, not been shattered, I would have continued in my old patterns. I would have tried to hold everything together in what I knew as "just the way it had to be held together" for me to be safe and successful. That veneer now lay in shards in every direction. What seemed and felt like destruction, was that cliché caterpillar or dragonfly transformation moment into the most incredible process of fun and discovery that continues to unfold to this very day. Join me as I share what I've discovered and have shared with so many others about the hidden potential that comes from discovering the wisdom of pain in our teaching. It can even be fun!

There's a Choice, Why Not Fun?

Supporting people living with chronic pain is heavy work. The work taxes the students who already have limited reserves because of their pain. Over time it can also drain us as professionals without care and proper intention/attention. That means there's a decision choice to be made by both parties (student and provider) as to how this work is to be framed. One choice is that this is a monster of heavy, exhausting work that seems invincible and unending (and that isn't a necessarily a false assessment). Another choice (with equal possibilities of being "true") is that this work, while heavy, holds the possibilities of being extremely meaningful and rewarding when approached with the intention of viewing the work as a potential opportunity for discovery and the innate "fun" of satisfying human curiosity through discovery. Both valid positions to start from, each with markedly different implications for being healing and sustainable for both parties.

We know from our chapters on yoga and pain that both intention and first-person narrative generate the physiological state of the individual (student *and* yoga professional). This physiological state sets the basic drives and awareness for the person. The choice between heavy work versus fun and discovery will generate a state. As with any other intention, it is expected you'll deviate and at times completely lose track of your intention. Self-compassion and a gentle chuckle with a back and forth shake of the head is your exercise to pull your wheels back up out of the old ruts of habit, resetting your course to resume your intention. This constant resetting continues a positive, self-reinforcing process creating the following benefits:

- Decreases the allostatic (stress) load to prime one for inquiry and discovery.

- Reduces fear and a sense of despair for student and provider alike.

- The celebration of incremental discoveries supports the autonomic nervous system.

- Each discovery reaches back to "edit" the self-story for the better prior to continuing forward.

- Evokes the delight of curiosity and further exploration generates momentum to continue.

- By reframing failures and setbacks as practices of self-compassion, this intention primes for further creativity by not looping into fear and failure narratives.

- Regular recollection of the steady flow of discoveries marks direction and progress in the journey, reinforcing both motivation and story.

Life is short and hard. I recommend choosing "fun and discovery" as a wise prescription for all of us. If you aren't sold yet, read on. If you are sold, then you are really going to love what follows.

> People who know how to creatively break the rules also know why the rules were there in the first place. They are not mere iconoclasts or rebels. (Rohr 2011, p.xxviii)

Modern Ills: Re-creation versus Distraction and Tedium

As you may recall from the pain, creativity, and wisdom chapters, you can now appreciate how each of us as human beings is an ongoing, self-creating process rather than some static structure and set of functions. Life in the big sense is constantly learning, adapting, and creating new possibles, as we also do in the miniature as individuals. This concept of ongoing re-creating has not been part of most people's understanding and certainly not part of the dominant Western culture. In fact, as Bateson attests, this systemic mutual learning (symmathesy) is extremely fluid and breaks us free from our self-centered, asmitâ world view that generates suffering according to the kleshas. Discovering these relationships of mutual learning (the opposite of separation/asmitâ) is yoga and a big part of what differentiates wisdom from mere knowledge.

Adopting this fundamental wisdom of the intimate interrelationships of all of reality invites participation, hope, and fascination. Shouldn't this be headlines on the TV news? Unfortunately, this perspective is in sharp contrast to what often becomes our modern lives of continuous distraction and the tedium of just enduring, without direction or hope for the future. This sounds like I'm just talking about the students. I'm not. I'm also pointing toward we yoga professionals. When our well runs dry or out of habit, we resort to teaching the same old stuff, possibly slightly tweaked, but it evokes a sense of tedium and sadness on our part. Maybe I should be writing this in the first person? I'm betting I'm not alone though. That same asmitâ orientation by us of being separate and cut off then pulls both us and our students into a state of weariness that accompanies the frenetic pace of society. On a good note, that weariness may have also led you to pick up this book (and me to write it). We all know there's got to be a better way to refresh our practice for all involved.

There is a better way. That way is grounded in the focus and the thrill of discoveries we make together, rather than me or you casting pearls of wisdom and corrective directions to our students. It is so easy to slip back into that doer mode that this statement bears repeating. When boredom and distraction arrive, see them as guides pointing you away from that asmitâ perspective and waving you back to the wisdom of symmathesy (mutual learning) and yoga. Over and over and over. A special bonus is this not only applies to your personal practice and teaching, but the very heart of your yoga business too. As we have noted, that unstruck sound you are to contribute to life is expressed from your heart space through your hands and voice. Let's take a minute to explore that essential relationship.

The Generative Heart of Your Business

Which business are we talking about? Our personal business practice or the larger business of our profession in general? Yes. Remember, how you perform your personal yoga practices affects how you arrive to teach, and how you teach and manage your business drives how you do your formal yoga practice. How that business exists in the community locally and as a thread in the larger yoga profession quite literally weaves the reality of yoga and yoga therapy in the world. That larger fabric then feeds back to how your role is perceived by current and future students and business clients. Endless, intertwined loops, not in a straight circular fashion, but back and forth, reaching ahead and linking behind and through. A powerful, but delicate, weave of learning, editing, and actions from new possibles. If your personal practice continues to be or becomes one of fun, discovery, and delight, your business will reflect that through how you teach, how you interact with students and colleagues, and what new programming you generate because of your shift in your personal practice.

Consider this exercise for yourself right now: Sense a rut in your personal yoga practice. Open yourself to a new way of sensing and approaching your current practice that generates a deeper, more aware practice where you can discover subtle, but significant shifts in yourself (see Chapter 7 on practice ahead and Butera and Elgelid (2017) for examples). What you will discover is that by changing a rut you are adjusting Halifax's six domains (discussed earlier), which gives you new insights and nurtures you in surprising ways. Additionally, you will begin to gain insight into some of your related business quandaries, because just one part of you doesn't change, the entire kaleidoscope of you changes. You might then discover, while teaching, that rather than directing every fine point during a class or individual session, you begin to drop your "doer" mode to invite insight and participation from your students as you go, riffing off one another's insights and discoveries, setting up many more new possibles. This can include literally sharing your own experiences from your personal practice at home, but also opening to their creating fresh insight to both their needs and experiences, with all of you reaping the benefits of this re-created practice you could never have sketched out in a lesson plan.

This enhanced process leads to students enthusiastically renewing memberships, but also evangelizing for you and bringing in new students like themselves, who are longing for relief and community. Soon you are adding another class and have interest from the students in a longer Saturday workshop too. You capture these fresh, enthused testimonials, sharing them through social media, that generates new interest and a call from the local radio station wanting to interview you with this exciting new approach to supporting students in pain. Oh, no! What did you do?!? A good problem. Head back to your mat and keep surrendering with freshness and intention to relieve your and your students' suffering. For much more on this harvesting the full potential from group classes, see Taylor (2006). For now, how is it such a small change could make such a large difference downstream? Let's weave together some more of what we've discussed so far to better understand the power of wisdom.

Giving Non-violent Fishing Lessons

That last example might seem improbable to many of you. I welcome your skepticism, but also invite you to remain open to the possibility that acting on what we're exploring will foster surprises for you and your students as well. Unlike the usual self-help blather of create your vision board, repeating your affirmation of success, and so on, in order to get to some predetermined outcome of your imagination, we are practicing ishvara pranidhana through this process. That is, neither you, me, or your students can predict what will in fact relieve our suffering now or prevent it in the future. If it were the case that we did know, and I certainly no longer trust myself to know what's best, we could toss that niyama practice of surrendering to the greater mystery right in the dumpster. But isn't it fascinating that this process of teaching from wisdom still involves many of the same practices advocated by the self-help gurus, but they rest on an entirely different premise of causality and control. That premise isn't on some interventionist deity moving things around on the Life game board for our benefit or as compensation for good behavior. Nor is the premise that we are the deity and can therefore direct the game board. It seems it's that darn middle way, somewhere between the two.

We began the book by redefining what yoga might be, how it's more a verb or adverb than a noun. With yoga as the "how" of relationship/connectedness, we directly approached the kleshas as sources of suffering. Key to this new understanding of yoga was the empowerment of the student to participate in the ongoing process, rather than directing and fixing their brokenness while forfeiting their power. Holding that new possibility of what yoga might be, we then explored how this new yoga fit in the fabric of both traditional wisdom teachings and the emerging new wisdom discoveries of today. That is, wisdom isn't some static collection, but a living, breathing expression of the ongoing creation underway in our known universe. Which by definition, makes us wisdom, not separate from or needing to acquire it as a commodity. That asmitâ of separateness is so persistent, creeping up everywhere.

Our journey into our very limited understanding of pain from both traditional and modern pain theory clearly illuminated the complex, interrelated nature of existence. Under the lens of emerging science the surety of what pain is has dissolved and is now considered an emergent process tied to more and more of every fabric of our lives and our environment. Asmitâ withers under continued discernment, but with it the certainty of our dominant pattern of seeking the "just right" prescription for relieving the related suffering. Coupling our new found understanding around yoga and wisdom, there was a natural next step in visiting creativity as the only way forward from pain.

Stepping up to this new self-image of us as wisdom allowed us to explore what we presently understand about creativity and how sharply that understanding contrasts with what creativity has been sold as historically and even today. This emergent phenomenon that never ceases or rests again is not separate from us or something we need acquire through the "X-steps to becoming creative" being sold today. There we explored concepts and practices that transformed our understanding of creativity. While creativity is unpredictable and resistant to controlling outcomes, the conditions that prime us for creativity just happens to reflect the known outcomes of our yoga practices. That "everything is connected" stuff actually has some utility. But to be so powerful, it must be very hard, right? Yes and no. That's where we are right now in this chapter.

To be a full participant in the co-creation of bringing forward the future new possibles is going to happen with or without our consent. I am making the pitch that setting an intention of discovery and fun will complement our participation while making lighter the very real hard work of being alive. That work includes the concepts we've shared about yoga therapy as a creative response to pain. Holding that intention and then participating is not only fun and a discovery adventure for us, but for those we serve as well. And because these skills and perspectives aren't mechanical prescriptions for fixing some particular problem X, they are life skills the student and we will have to address whatever surprises emerge in the future. That teaching someone to fish versus giving them a fish thing. That's real empowerment that is incorporated (brought into the corpus/body) into society through each of our individual participation. We can only image-ine (create an image) of what that will lead to down the road.

We Are the Systems

There's a tendency to blame the systems for our challenges. However, in Chapter 2 we described the modern day systems theory of interdependency and how we are the systems, like it or not. Further, in order to change large systems (organizations, businesses, governments, multinationals) the most effective method is the personal practices of transformation and change of each individual in the larger system. Now there's real empowerment. And responsibility. Again this calls us to break out of the asmitâ-perspective of our own personal and professional practices. What we are sharing doesn't stop inside the "skin and skulls" of those we teach.

The effects of the ripple travel in unimagined ways literally around the globe. Recall my Minnesota story that has a former small-town Midwest physical therapist writing a book on yoga for a British publisher. My teacher, Jeff Wright, a high school special education instructor, drove 30 minutes weekly to teach a handful of us at our health club. Last month I was named to the Integrative Healthcare Policy Consortium's Task Force on Chronic Pain and Opioid Abuse as the yoga representative for the USA. Who saw that coming? The task force interfaces with agencies and policy makers to create the future of care in the USA. I'm "all in" that my personal practice might be important. So is yours and that of everyone you serve. We just don't know and certainly can't predict. We just practice with the surrender of ishvara pranidhana. Speaking of practice, why, that brings us to the next chapter. Are you ready? Let's go!

7

. . .

Practice Makes Possibles

Finally, the "how to" for transforming your way of supporting students and yourself by teaching yoga therapy for pain as a creative response. The wisdom, of course, emerges as we've discovered to generate new possibles à la Kaufman. Those new possibles invite you take new actuals into action to enable the next generation of new possibles and so on. In yoga, of course, we call this practice (origin Greek *praktikos* or practical work). Theory is nice, but practice that leads to practical work is where we are now. First, we will review some general guidelines for you and your students, then progress through a series of actions or exercises to prime for the next creative response. Following these guidelines and creating new practices fosters the empowerment for both you and your students as defined in the definition of yoga therapy, "the process of empowering individuals to progress toward." Were this a simple recipe prescription from me, then how would you and those you serve be empowered to respond to the inevitable pains ahead? So we begin to practice keeping in mind that creativity requires both the surprise of the insight and the practice of techniques per Bruner (1997). Deliberate effort is the fuel to fire creativity… And so, the fun of discovery begins!

What Will Your Starting Practice Be?

Taking new action as yoga professionals includes literally doing things quite differently than you did before. More often, though, using what you've read so far will probably have you doing the very same movements but now in a very different frame of mind and intention. On video your day may look the same, as generally the "how" changes more than the "what" of your actions. There will be times the "what" changes, especially as your skills expand and new possibles are generated, but chances are, on the surface, at least initially, there won't be huge visible changes as much of this material is "inside" work.

I do invite you to be bold, but not obnoxious, in trying on new practices and the actions that emerge from practicing. By bold, I mean addressing one or more deep seated patterns, not externally behaving brashly or in an overbearing manner. As a guideline though, consider how stealth can you be around your changes? If you do this correctly, your engagement isn't to make you look better or radically different, but to transform the moment of suffering you are sharing with the other. When you boldly, but gently alter your past response, it may be tortuous on your insides as the urge to not change is very powerful. However, if you sustain awareness with presence, and the intention to empower the other rather than leave them dependent as in past practice, you and your students will both be empowered in the process.

Starting small is probably the best advice. One new action today and watch. Then repeat again the next day. Biting off too much change is difficult for your own personal system and really hard for the larger external systems to accept, to include students with chronic pain. You have the rest of your life to do this, remember? Like they often say about yoga, this process of creativity is slow medicine, but strong medicine. Just be sure to take some every day.

Finally, adopt the integral "both/and" way of being, *and* be aggressive (not just small and gentle). Give things time to emerge, but also ruthlessly discard what your embodied perception guides you to eliminate. Consider these new practices as rapid learning experiments that are bound to be modified and changed regularly. Schedule regular reappraisals of your practices that show weak or no results. Move on to some new action, but garner the learning that came from reflecting on the effort anyway. There'll always be some insight. (More on this at the end of the chapter.) This section will be written as it applies to you a yoga professional, but presume most, if not all the practices can be applied to those you serve as well. Let's adapt an easy sense of humor about us not being so all-important or responsible, and enjoy these experiments in life.

Create a Workspace

Set a time each week when you will review your week and plan the coming week. As I mentioned in Chapter 5 on creativity, I personally like David Allen's embodied approach of *Getting Things Done* (2002). The book details the actions that are involved during this 20–30-minute review and, without this regular pause to reflect, the change process slows in a hurry. This single recurring action generates momentum that fuels effective new insights and actions for you. Like any process, it takes a good deal of effort to initiate the habit, but once underway it will be a force to drive many innovative actions for you in the future. As we discussed in creativity, something must be destroyed to make room on your calendar for this new weekly workspace. Be ruthless, but in a ahimsic (non-harming) kind of way.

Capture Your Ideas

New insights and ideas will begin to emerge, often at the oddest times. Create a method for how you are going to capture new ideas in a way that assures you know you won't lose them. Again, Allen (2002) has a great variety of simple systems for this process. For those with smartphones there is the notepad app, audio recorder, email/text the idea to yourself…virtually an endless list of options to include the classic little black notepad in your pocket or purse. Choose what fits you and start capturing. You will be surprised how quickly capturing new insights becomes a regular occurrence. It's my favorite collection.

Set an Embodied Action Schedule

To fulfill our intention to act, we move from our bodies. But of course, right? Well most planning systems fail to take that fact into account.

Most systems have you list all your goals and subtasks and then schedule them. What isn't considered is you need to be physically in the right circumstance to complete the action (i.e., "Visit mom" is on Saturday but you are at soccer tournament that day). Allen's (2002) book details more but, suffice it to say, you need to plan where you literally will be physically and what actions you can take there. I know this seems obvious, but reflect back on some task you've been meaning to complete and notice if your physical locale wasn't part of what has prevented you from completing the task. An embodied system assures you will be physically in the proper environment to act, setting you up for the "asana" of action. The system you devise should also have a reliable way of notifying you of deadlines before it's too late to act accordingly. Such a notification process releases you from that nagging neurophysiological tension of "Isn't there something I should be doing?" and creates more space per the first practices that follow. This may sound complicated, but it is far simpler than it sounds and Allen (2002) has great ways to do so, especially with email. Did you order it yet?

Seek Feedback on New Actions

Asking for feedback makes us vulnerable to criticism. Yet feedback is exactly what we need to better discern the quality and skillfulness of our action, not unlike teacher cues in asana. When you have tried something new (i.e., asking a student to share more, when in the past you might have passed a comment off as too messy to pursue) let the other person know that this was new for you and seek their response as to whether they found the new action helpful or not. Either way, ask specifically in what way it was or wasn't helpful. This feedback process models for the student new ways of behaving from vulnerability themselves and brings you both to a more peer-level, mutual learning team model of our complex being. Use the feedback then to inform your next round of action and enhance your skill in action.

You should also access your own feedback on actions. I don't mean just thinking, "Did that turn out like I intended?" Rather, sit quietly sensing your breath pattern. Once you sense an even pattern, gently ask yourself about the new action in question, "What did I discover in this new action?", and then continue to experience your breath pattern, noting any changes or shifts. If it remains steady or even softens, there's a good chance you sense safety and satisfaction around the new action. If there's a significant shift or alteration in the pattern, stay with the breath and notice if some insight or new perspective might emerge from the stillness. Remember, we are wisdom and we become wise through both internal communication *and* community interaction. This feedback from both sources sets the new possibles for the next action, hopefully generating a new actual that eases more of the suffering as intended.

Gather a Cadre to Support New Action

Building off the importance of community feedback, recruiting a cadre (skilled workforce) of people who have the experience and skills you lack to attain your goals is crucial. Your effectiveness will soar when you limit yourself to doing what you do well or can learn to do well, and seek out support for those things you can't do or do inefficiently. I've wasted countless hours trying to do things that could have been done better and more efficiently out of pride, scarcity, ignorance, and just being cheap! Save yourself the suffering. To assemble this cadre, sit down and plan what resources and skills are needed to support a new action. The first few times will, of course, be somewhat clumsy as a new action for you, but repetition will make it natural and often automatic. List the personnel or skill sets based on the size of your project and the identified work ahead. Then assign responsibilities accordingly, bringing in those additional people for the work you have identified. Notice any resistance, reassess if necessary, and then breathe your way into it as you would in a new asana engagement. Failure to address this basic conflict of avoiding this step implementing something new is almost guaranteed to create future suffering for someone. Like you?

Note that when you honestly assess what additional members you need to bring in as a cadre, that invites the actions of establishing new relationships beyond your silo of your experience. So, ask for help and extend your network of contacts and interests with confidence. This new wider net of connections primes the emergence for effective surprises down the road. People want to help as a rule, so ask for the help you need as you build your team. I needed 15 contributing authors for an earlier book I wrote and edited. Only one person I invited flat out refused, and one other couldn't because of other commitments but sent me to someone that could. Granted I did the legwork of vetting those I didn't personally know first. That extra bit of work building my cadre led to a 100 percent on-time completion of chapters. Building your various cadres will be time well spent as you assemble implementation teams, to include just marshalling your own internal team of resources for personal projects. Don't create alone. Yoke with those that can best deliver on your well-intended new actions.

Yoga Was an Oral Tradition: Become a Good Storyteller

In this era of information overload there's a temptation to be information "dumpers." In one class or private instruction we tell ourselves, "I must share all the new pain science, the science of creativity, the history of yoga, and its neurophysiological correlates, and on and on." Can you feel it? We have mentioned story many times so far in this book. Gottschal summed up storytelling perfectly when he wrote:

> The storytelling mind is allergic to uncertainty, randomness, and coincidence. It is addicted to meaning. If the storytelling mind cannot find meaningful patterns in the world, it will try to impose them. In short, the storytelling mind is a factory that churns out true stories when it can, but will manufacture lies when it can't. (2012, p.102)

Given that power, think about the teachers or therapists in your life who have been most effective. How did they teach and reach you most effectively? Chances are they told great stories. Up until very recently that is how yoga was taught too. That's what we humans do. We tell each other stories and the best storytellers can inspire entire cultures and epochs. In the medical science this "lowest form of evidence" (anecdotal) has been denigrated over the past century. However, the very same research literature is revealing that this is what students' value and that good stories (aka student narratives and our student education stories) affect the outcome of our teaching. Therefore, study the art and science of storytelling. Storytelling is a skill that requires practice.

This art and science begins, and includes, that constant story going on within yourself. From that listening to self-practice, then begin to listen more deeply to other's stories. Once you've really heard the other's story, and have listened to your own to be sure of your intention, when it's appropriate, offer gentle, or not so gentle, edits of your and their story. When your story moves both the heart and mind of others, it will surpass any other yoga tool on your belt. Every storyteller can improve and my re-editing of this paragraph the past 30 minutes I hope is proof.

From now on, pay close attention to how stories influence you and gain insight upon reflection on those stories. Then use those insights to improve your stories in your yoga instruction. For example, read and feel this single sentence story about compassion, "Having felt he'd been heard, his chest gently unfurled as his eyes brightened with the dawning awareness" versus "His posture improved with a visible chest opening." Boring! Whereas the first is powerful and visceral as you can feel that same experience echo within you, can't you? Additionally, the cadre-building in the exercise above will be more successful if you are a good storyteller to get people to sign on, and then you will need an even better story for them to stay on, as the work gets underway. And I'm telling you a story right now by the way. Has my story moved you to craft your storytelling skills differently in the future?

Act: Loose That Arrow Arjuna

Our habit is to try to push from the mental into action. This exercise invites us to enact new actions from engagement to shift the mental, and do it sooner rather than later. Breaking free of our patterns/samskara requires overcoming inertia in our habits, both habits of mind and bodily action. We now understand from the bidirectional nature of the bodymind that the body can drive the mental and vice versa. Courage isn't feeling no fear, but feeling the fear and acting anyway. In the practices that follow, developing your affective attunement and insight will prime you to be able to engage sooner in new actions and learn faster from the feedback you gain. So we draw back, take aim, and then loose our arrow of new action. The result is beyond our control but opens the next emerging new possibles. Discernment/Action: the work of the yoga professional. Over and over and over.

karmaṇy-evādhikāras te mā phaleṣhu kadāchana
mā karma-phala-hetur bhūr mā te saṅgo 'stvakarmaṇi

karmani—in prescribed duties; *eva*—only; *adhikāraḥ*—right; *te*—your; *mā*—not; *phaleṣhu*—in the fruits; *kadāchana*—at any time; *mā*—never; *karma-phala*—results of the activities; *hetuḥ*—cause; *bhūḥ*—be; *mā*—not; *te*—your; *saṅgaḥ*—attachment; *astu*—must be; *akarmaṇi*—in inaction

Translation:

Bhagavad Gita 2.47: You have a right to perform your prescribed duties, but you are not entitled to the fruits of your actions. Never consider yourself to be the cause of the results of your activities, nor be attached to inaction.

Ouch! The Teacher Has Arrived

As each new "ouch" in life arrives, literal or metaphoric, see if you can welcome its arrival as your next teacher. Trying on new actions and creating what hasn't been is guaranteed to be messy and prickly along the way. Reframing those "ouches" from bad to teachers will modify your stories, invite space for discernment, and they happen often. And that's OK. Think of it as your engaged pratyahara practice as you pause to sense with reduced reaction, and then respond creatively. Continuing your conventional yoga practice and engaging in what follows here will make that formerly nasty knocking of pain at your door transform over time. Jump in and watch the emergence.

As you read through the following practices, highlight those that capture your attention. Select one space making practice and 2–3 other practices to begin under the guidelines above. Set realistic goals of your intention for doing the practice, when you will do it, how frequently, and for how long.

Please Note

Remember implementing new actions is the harder half of innovation (the new idea being the easier half). So rather than strive, relax into your improvisations. Keep a ready sense of humor along the way. Remember all our efforts are quite hilarious when viewed from a distance, just teetering between Greek comedy and tragedy, so don't take things too seriously.

Then watch how your internal and external worlds are transformed in the co-emergent creative process and enjoy the ride.

Making Space for Silence Exercises

We begin these practices with an invitation to silence. Silence is a key capacity to cultivate and it is from silence that so often effective surprises emerge for us and those we teach. Our Western culture is very biased to "doing" first as both a value and as part of the violence of our historic systems we described in Chapter 3. Our age of uncertainty hints at the wisdom of restoring balance between the states of doing and of being/ silence. Let us first consider this rationale, then follow up with practices to engage and explore silence in preparation for the remaining practices. These making space exercises are only a few of the many practices and are not intended to be an exhaustive treatment of the topic of silence. That would be another book.

How do you create environments that will prime you and those you serve to generate creative, yogic practices that lead to reduced suffering? As you begin, remember you move together *with* your students, no longer leading ahead as the expert. You will want to welcome the silence of "not knowing" as it arises, remembering there is no need to hurry to fill the silence with activity or "certainty." Rather, with the student, you will begin in a spirit of exploration, compassion, and deep caring, knowing your innate individual and collective creativity will emerge. In that act of knowing, healing occurs as our lives contribute to the new possibles that birth the next actuals.

It is important that before attempting to generate alternative approaches and good questions as forms of self-discovery of wisdom's *oneself*, you embark on more clearly seeing who you think you are and, in seeing yourself, *understand* what your assumptions really are, as those assumptions are what blind us to many new possibles. This making space section is not just from a "head-oriented" conceptual thinking about your and your students' assumptions. These approaches will allow you to more deeply explore the assumptions, and how those assumptions create limited perspectives. Often when exploring new approaches to practice you can experience reactions to your existing practices. These reactions will define new perspectives in opposition to what was your normal way of being and teaching in the world. This is another process of deconstructing, or making space, as the "destruction as the first step of creativity." Slowly the practices will examine what in the past may have been bricks of certainty. Through these practices and inquiry, you will literally transform your knowing to allow new possibles to arise from the generated experience of the Silence that is always present behind the noise of our habits.

Additionally, these making space practices are important for your smaller, local ordinary creativity to emerge for yourself. The space made will offer an important foundation for your teaching both individual and group yoga in contrast to the normal crush of so much activity. We will address later in this chapter how the practices take on even greater importance at the community and institutional levels of change I've advocated for in Chapters 2 and 5. Our efforts at those wider levels of connection to initiate creativity priming without first considering the many differences in assumptions between all the parties participating in change initiatives is bound to fail. Silence gained in these making space exercises can allow us to slow down and gain insights into the "differences that make a difference" that we would otherwise rush past in a habitual doing mode. This will be especially evident when you begin to move from the former "I'm the expert" yoga-related programs created by you the teacher to creating together with the students or organization as a collaborative team. More on that later.

How do we begin to make space? By deconstruction of certainty. There will be other deconstructing exercises further into the chapter, but these first few will begin to bring down the unseen walls of certainty we hold onto so tightly. Adopting new ways of seeing (metaperspectives) is necessary for us to correct misperceptions (vrittis). This clarity brings new understanding and discernment that prime us for expressing our creativity as both individuals and within our communities of interconnected humans. These deconstructing practices will begin to release your habitual singular views that have limited your understanding and generated at best, only a partial, if not inaccurate, foundation from which to create. Said another way, in order to construct, you and your students must hone your skills to be able to deconstruct or unlearn. After the deconstructions, there will be some simple, embodied practices to bring even more space that can be realized via additional somatic, mental, and emotional quieting practices.

The following practices are meant to be experienced as a complex, interwoven whole, rather than as a linear prescription of activities one following the other. You can begin anywhere in these exercises. Take your time. Do them rather than just reading about them, please. You can return to them once you have completed the book to revise your plan of what mix might be best for your circumstance and goals as time flows. The only structure I would advocate would be to begin and end each practice with creating some space for silence very deliberately. (Caution: Don't dispense any of these practices before practicing them several times for yourself, because it is so hard to teach what we don't know.)

Any practice that you plan to incorporate, just jot IWFD vertically and next to each letter note:

Your Intention: _____

When will I do it: _____

How Frequently: _____

For this long/Duration (repetitions/time/days): _____

First, What's There?

Living simply, or eliminating clutter, is a popular self-help topic today. The pitch is typically that by clearing your external clutter you will make space and then feel better. As yoga professionals, we can smile and appreciate that, yes, external environment plays a role in how we feel, but if you've made it this far in the book, you have an understanding that it's probably the clutter within that generated the clutter without, right? So, this first exercise is to take an inventory of our internal junk drawer, spare bedroom, attic, or garage where we have stored our stuff.

Get comfortable, pull out some paper to write down your answers (don't just think them), write without filtering, and most of all, have fun deconstructing your reality.

1. Reconsider your view of yoga and health: What is the matter with yoga and the health of your community in general now? What matters to you most in both? What is fun? What tires you?

What would make you spring out of bed in the morning about yoga and health? What part of your personal or business practice needs its own yoga care? What parts of your yoga skills could be better utilized to change you and those you serve for better health?

2. Reconsider the form and function of what you can control. What things do you do out of obligation, but not inspiration? Why? Could they be done differently? Could technology, delegation, or innovation change any of what you do control? Dig deep into the tiniest details from how you greet students or friends first thing to how you say farewell to your most difficult student. Pick through a mental video of your entire day, pulling out single frames and asking, what assumptions drive this behavior/technique or process? No activity is sacrosanct.

3. Take account of what tools you have beyond yoga skills boundaries. List all the talents, passions, and abilities you have that are not being utilized in your current business or life practice. Yes, your ability to doodle cartoon faces, make the best pickled onions, or arrange flowers…no filters, list them all.

4. Bring systems thinking to yoga. Sketch out the interconnections of all the systems you can think of that affect you, your work environment, your students, their communities, and so on. Just write them in a circle and start linking them with lines, multidirectional arrows to the others, creating a huge web/yoke of the complexity of the human experience knowing it is only a weak mechanical rendering à la Nora Bateson. So the messier the better. There's nothing to do with this but keep a running tab on it over a couple of weeks as you tear down and discover new relationships to add to the sketch.

5. Re-establish faith in and the use of relationship/connectedness as what matters most in yoga. Oh no, the yoga shadow! Scary stuff, but we must. What have you been told about yoga that says otherwise that something else is most important? Is it true? When do you have the most rewarding experiences at your business? What do students say mattered most to them? Who comes back to say thanks and what is it they thank you for? If you were going

to be bold and audacious in your use of connectedness, what would you start doing differently tomorrow? If you struggled thinking of things for this exercise or the next, ask those you live and work with for their input. If they're honest, they can show you what you missed.

6. Remember, embrace and celebrate loving kindness. Like the last exercise, but also grounded in our working definition of creativity being tied to compassion: for self and the other. What things do you do now that aren't rooted in loving kindness? Could they be changed, and, if so, how? What things are rooted? What could you do more of to show loving kindness? Why wouldn't you? Have you surrendered control of some of this to someone or some authority that doesn't warrant it? What would it feel like, and more importantly, what would it look like to live more from a sense of celebrating loving kindness?

Find an old file and put your answers in there for your eyes only. Cycle back to this exercise again as new insights emerge or real world encounters add to your lists. Having gone through the clutter to become aware of much of it, we can trust our innate integration to begin to resolve and organize as emergent new possibles. The next exercise is not to squint your brow and line up the parts to fix. Just the opposite in fact. "Soften your forehead," as I often heard Swami Veda Bharati say. And dive into the following.

Rotation of Consciousness

Now we shift our attention from the relatively very heady, conceptual work of inventorying thoughts, fears and desires, to experiencing and resting in our embodied state. If some of the "clutter" shows up as a memory/thought/image, notice it, and come back to the directions below of sensing, leaving the clutter for later with a soft smile.

Assume a comfortable supine or seated position with your back straight and supported and your eyes closed. Your feet should be on the ground, knees slightly wider than hip-width apart, and hands resting softly on your lap or thighs in sitting or at your side supine. This somatic awareness exercise will be familiar to most readers and quiets the central nervous system while enhancing bodily perception to make space for new awareness.

Starting with your right thumb, name that body part silently to yourself, then sense that part without moving it, then move to each finger on the right hand, wrist, forearm, and so on up the arm. From the right shoulder move your attention down the side of the right trunk, naming ribs, abdomen, back, front of the hip, and so forth all the way down the front of the right leg and across the toes, then back up the sole of the foot and the back of the leg naming/sensing each area. Once done on the right, repeat on the left side of the body. After the left side is finished, then do the same for the right side of the head, being very detailed, and then the left side of the head, finishing with sensing your entire body. Rest several minutes in the silence that follows, keeping your attention directed to just feeling the soft, natural sensations of your resting breath.

After opening your eyes, if you had any insights, emotional responses, or other ideas that aren't easily categorized, jot some notes for your folder to archive the experience.

Alternate Nostril Breathing...the Balanced Breath

Most of you will know this simple breathing exercise and it can be done in the same positions as the Rotation of Consciousness. By alternating not only your attention from one side to the other, but also experiencing the related sensations of filling, temperature change, and vibration this practice has a deep, documented quieting effect on the central nervous system.

Start with just 2–3 minutes, and gradually add a minute every couple of sessions. The breath should be natural, neither pushing or pulling the breath faster or harder. The rules are beginning with an inhalation in the left nostril, switch to the other nostril every time you are filled with breath, and when finishing do so on a left nostril exhalation.

- Cover right nostril with an index finger, inhale left nostril.

- Switch finger to close left, exhale out of right nostril.

- Inhale right, switch finger to close right nostril.

- Exhale left nostril.

- Inhale left, switch finger to close right nostril, and so on.

After you finish, sit quietly for a couple minutes paying attention to your experience with your eyes closed. Can you sense the spaciousness/silence created by the practice? Do you feel bigger or smaller? Is your awareness focused or diffuse? When you open your eyes, record any impressions or experiences for your folder.

Focused Breathing

Quite simply, sustained focus and redirection of attention to these tasks makes it very difficult to sustain attention on the clutter. The repetitive vibration/sensation of the breath are known to inhibit the self-referential portions of the brain, generating a sense of expansion and connection within the experience of a deep silence.

- Gently rest tip of tongue on the center of the roof of your mouth.

- Mouth closed: Breathe in and out of the nose naturally without pushing or pulling the breath, keeping tongue connected, but soft.

- Imagery: Imagine breathing "through" the tongue…both on the in and out breath.

- Repeat for 3–5 minutes, eyes stay soft.

After completing, rest again and note your perceptions of change in the amount of silence and spaciousness you are experiencing. Then mindfully open your eyes and record any insights or experiences you may have had for your folder.

Soham Mantra

I'm often surprised to learn how few yoga professionals actually practice mantram. As you know, the repetition of a sound, even just imagining the sound without audibly making it, creates deep quieting of the central nervous system. Choose your favorite or use the mantra of Soham, a Sanskrit term meaning "I am that" as a simple but powerful tool for staying present to the moment. When used this way, "Soham" serves to control one's breathing pattern, as in focused breathing above, to help achieve a deeper, natural breath, and to gain concentration as the clutter falls away.

- Sooooo…is the sound of inhalation, and is remembered in the mind along with that inhalation.

- Hahmmmm…is the sound of exhalation, and is remembered in the mind along with that exhalation.

- Repeat for three minutes or so. Then for one minute do only the "ham" on the exhale, remaining silent on the inhale.

- Then stay silent on both the inhale and exhale for one minute.

After completing, rest again and note your perceptions of change in the amount of silence and spaciousness you are experiencing. Then mindfully open your eyes and record any insights or experiences you may have had for your folder.

Concluding Making Space Comments

While these first exercises were written for your practice, as you can see they are easily adapted for your students to perform as part of the making space. The intention and focus can be scaled down to reflect the students' specific circumstances, or merely redirected toward their vocation and passion.

The Practices

Now that you and they have begun to sweep clean some space, it is time to move on to exercises. These noncreative practices (remembering we *are* creativity, these practices merely prime us to allow that innate creativity to emerge) invite new behaviors, new anatomy, and physiology in us via learning and neuroplasticity, and ultimately, out of this silence, each of our collective futures will emerge. Have fun, dabble as you are attracted and note especially those activities from which you or your students are repelled or dismissive. As you probably already teach, very often the resistance or avoidance to a practice is a signal for pointing you to exactly to what might most radically prime you to transform your life and the lives that you encounter in life. Obviously, you would have first screened for and asked about triggers related to trauma or other related risk factors.

I'm presuming you will continue your usual yoga practice. The following practices have been selected because most are not conventional yoga practices. I will leave the instruction of conventional practices to the many fine references that already exist in the market. I have artificially divided these practices into our chapter topics for organization. We all know this division is arbitrary by the integral nature of our being, but it gives our minds a comfortable skeleton of organization from which to set off in exploration.

Yoga Practices

Asana Ahimsâ? At your next class or practice, observe and work with all of the emotions and moods that arise. Do you experience anger at your body? Do you work your body with the frustrations of your day and then expect your body to do what you want? The cultivation of a soft spaciousness of body and mind ought to be the intention of yoga. Create your intention as you go onto your mat, then reflect on your experience as you leave the mat. Make it a ritual of practice, opening and closing by honoring non-harming.

The Art of Inwardness: In your personal yoga practice and for your students, adopt the pedagogy (teaching style) of interiority. Many of us do to some degree, but encourage even more development and exploration into new ways for yourself and others. Also, offer ways to extend the interior focus off the mat in daily life. In our outward directed society, there's little risk most would overdo this exercise. The art within is a treasure to behold as our eye of interiority sharpens and develops.

Fearing Compassion? That's no joke. We do. Here some scales to download and complete with scoring instructions: https://compassionatemind.co.uk/uploads/files/fears-of-compassion-scale.pdf; read the supporting article (Gilbert *et al.* 2011). Go ahead, nothing to fear here.

Wisdom Practices

Meet Judgment, Cynicism, and Fear: These three characters derail our best wisdom practices, so it is worthwhile to learn to sense and recognize their presence from an embodied awareness. You might notice that judgments use the door behind your eyebrows, while cynicism (that'll never work, we tried that before, etc.) hangs back behind the heart area generally, and then notice when fear shows up. Fear is frequently lounging in the guts, often lower than higher. Try keeping a bodymap and, when any of these three come knocking, note where they like to hang out. The more skilled you become as sensing, the less error and inaccuracy in your insights!

M. C. Bateson LOVE Exercise: Mary Catherine Bateson defines love as "the ability to value a difference in another AND find something in common" (2017). The next time you or your student has the experience of dislike or distaste for another or a group, stop, pause, and ask, "What can I value that is different for them and what do we have in common?" Notice what changes and practice as needed.

Between-ness Muscle Pumping: It is a skill to be able to sense our connections to things outside our bodies. Our society is extremely deconditioned in this regard. Rest assured, though, if you steadily attempt to develop your sense, perception, and perhaps ultimately awareness of connections or between-ness of your mind outside your skin, your ability will improve. Attention and intention will drive the workout, coupled with sensing through embodiment so many connections never before attended to by you or your student. It feels good too, no muscle burn in this workout, just a nice rep every time you notice a between-ness. Pump it up.

Four Streams of Awareness: Siegel describes those streams as SOCK: Sensing, Observing, Conceptualizing, and Knowing (2017, p.231). Sharpen your skill to see if you can differentiate each experience *and* link them into integration. Can you sense each separately? Can you allow two or more to merge together and yet have a sense of each property despite not being separate? Start small with just two and be patient. Most of all, have fun.

Symmathesy Exercise: First, allow complexity to come forward. Next, pause the impulse to find the cause. Then ask, what might increase mutual learning within the situation you have identified. Do any previously unseeable possibilities appear? Now repeat the five steps indefinitely (N. Bateson 2017, p.116).

Learning to Learn: Life's questions do not have answers. Nora Bateson (2017, p.142) writes there are, however, "avenues where inquiry is invited." With practice and luck this practice will lead to further inquiries. Our goal is to ask good questions in hopes they lead to better questions. She further cautions that a simple question gets a simple answer, and we do not live in a simple world. The steps to remember when learning to learn: (1) We cannot know the systems, but we can know more; (2) We cannot perfect the systems, but we can do better; (3) The evolution of our own ability to understand and interact with the world around us is an increase in our ability to be sensitive to information we have previously been blind to and then ask better questions; and (4) Repeat without end.

Landscaping: Remember you are part of the landscape, poet John O'Donohue (2017) urged. When you come out of your house, notice if you are walking into an inanimate geographical location, merely put there for you to get to a destination, or whether you are emerging out into a landscape that is just as much, if not more, alive as you, but in a totally different form. If you go toward the landscape with an open heart and a sincere, watchful reverence, he believes that you will be absolutely amazed at what it will reveal to you. Landscape isn't just matter, but it is actually alive. Stop and notice. Can you sense how landscape recalls you into a mindful mode of stillness, solitude, and silence, where you can truly receive time and being in your life?

Find the Pattern That Connects: Gregory Bateson used "the pattern that connects," knowing it is a phrase difficult to understand. Is there a pattern that is "findable" as a code that can be discovered and understood (has form)? Or is "the pattern that connects" acknowledging the constant change which takes place in ways that go beyond our culture's customary styles of reasoning (the process)? This paradox of seeing "the pattern that connects" as both process and form is your exercise as an observer, to expand your integrative capacity. Can you see both the form and process involved between you and the surface you are sitting on? How about between you and the reader/book you are using? It's there. Can you find both?

Time the Thief: We've become the victim and target of time. It runs us instead of us running it. When we make time to be still and with ourselves, then our being can catch up and bring forward what has been transforming in us. This is O'Donohue's "secret work" that we call emergence. Such pauses generate a threshold, over which we can then step into the next moment. No pause, no secret work and no threshold… just headlong racing a clock. Pause. Let the threshold emerge. Then, with great awareness, step through on your time.

Introduction to Cartography (Map Drawing): In science, we have been told, things need to be measured and weighed. But relationships cannot be measured and weighed; relationships need to be mapped. Thus the perceptual shift from objects to relationships goes hand in hand with a change of methodology from measuring to mapping. When we map relationships, we find certain configurations that occur repeatedly. These are what we call patterns. Networks, cycles, and boundaries are examples of patterns of organization that are characteristic of living systems and are at the center of attention in systems science. Anytime you find yourself in awe or confusion, roll out a fresh sheet of paper and begin to map. No pressure, because maps aren't reality, just tools more or less useful for navigating reality. Better maps, better understanding and insight.

Are Those Rose-Colored Lens? To quote Heisenberg (1958, p.58): "What we observe is not nature itself, but nature exposed to our method of questioning." Thus systems thinking involves a shift from objective to "epistemic" science, to a framework in which epistemology—"the method of questioning"—becomes an integral part of scientific theories and how we experience our reality. Make yourself a series of make-believe lens to swap on and off like picking out new glasses. One from a serious scientist, another a small child in wonder, another a dying elder, etc. Create a variety of lens and watch life change before your very eyes based on your lens. Then practice using them in all you do and experience.

Contemplation: Our learned, dualistic thinking can get us only so far, per Rohr (2013). We need new software code for processing the really big questions, such as death, love, infinity, suffering, and God.

Contemplation is a non-dualistic way of seeing the moment. Originally, contemplation was simply prayer, the practice of living in the right now, the present moment. Being contemplative, he says, will teach us how to actually experience our experiences, whether good, bad, or ugly, and how to let those experiences transform us. Be careful of words (thought and speech), because by themselves they invariably divide the moment; pure presence lets it be what it is, as it is. When you can be present to all that arrives, and drop the labels and stories when they arise, you are in contemplation. He suggests that the exercise can begin by reading an excerpt from a sacred text or sitting the presence of beauty to prime for a contemplative state. Contemplate that.

Pain Practices (Yikes!)

Navigating Stimuli Exercise: Noticing stimuli and directing attention are the core of yoga, as I wrote very early in the book. Of course, we can easily make the simple complex by directing our attention to discover that there are many types of stimuli. Classical yoga texts note many types of stimuli: the five senses; disease; dullness; doubt; negligence; laziness; dissipation secondary to craving; delusion; lack of concentration; instability/restlessness; suffering/frustration; and disturbed breathing. Our practice then is to "wake up" to notice if our attention is directed toward anyone of these stimuli. Once we notice, then we have a set of new possibles because we can choose to redirect our attention elsewhere. That choice creates a new actual, along with a new assessment of where attention is now, new choice, same or new direction. Over and over. May seem obvious to a yoga professional on a certain level. To the person with chronic pain, I find it is of enormous relief to assume the power of attention directing. The practice does require patience and repetition, but the associated freedom from being "stuck" is a big gift. Have a safe trip navigating.

Remapping or Updating Your GPS Resolution: While we are on the travel theme, keeping our modern day global positioning map (GPS) updated is key to navigate with ease and efficiency. An old map, or one that is corrupted, creates suffering on the road. Those smudged or corrupted sensory and motor maps/representations we described in the pain chapter need "refreshing" or updating just like the apps in our devices and vehicles. How do humans do that? Attention to stimuli of course, with the more modes (tactile, visual, and auditory) the better. When we invite students to attend to alignment, sensation, mirrored visual feedback, appropriate verbal and tactile cues, prop support, and so on, it is helpful to suggest that, in paying attention, they are updating their mapping system. One fun way is to have them do an asana to one side, pause back in a neutral position, sense the feelings/dimensions/qualities of the first side compared to the unattended side. Then complete the second side and reassess both sides, noting the "updates" and changes in quality and resolution. Bad map, long trip. Good map, happy traveling. Update regularly.

The PAIN Exercise: An acronym from Christine Wolf, MD for:

> *P*utting kindness toward self and others into the mix
>
> *A*llowing experience to be there, just as it is
>
> *I*nquiring with interest into physical sensations, emotions, or thoughts
>
> *N*ot identifying with the pain. Stop asking "Why is this happening to me?" Instead, remember it's a natural process. (Wolf 2015)

This practice helps to shift the locus of control from the outside ("this is happening to me and there is nothing I can do about it") to the inside ("this is happening to me but I can choose how I relate to it"). Note how this is another attention and narrative rewriting and redirecting practice with an easy to remember acronym: PAIN.

Holy Holons: Holons are the relationships of symmathesies and systems. I am a human body. I'm composed of multiple systems, which are made up of organs, tissues, cells, organelles, and so on. I am also a part of a family, neighborhood, community, state, country, hemisphere, planet, and so on. Now list some of your holons: Note where there is any pain or suffering at any of the levels and how that affects other levels. What are the stimuli that let you know there is pain or suffering there? Do those stimuli have any gaps where new learning or action might affect the level of the holon and therefore other related levels? How would a happier holon look? What are you going to do to create gaps between stimuli to create new possibles? Often the opportunity for change lies in the holons above or below, versus where we habitually focus our attention. The same is even more the case for those with chronic pain. Teach 'em holons.

Graded Movement Exploration: Movement, as we've explored, lies along a very different and rich spectrum than just a part moving through space. We talked about how thoughts are movements. That movements have intention and are not valueless, random changes in space. There are good resources for learning the principles of graded movement in Chapter 4. If you haven't been exposed to the process, seek out training or purchase some guides. The information is critical as you choose to offer movement-based learning. When you explore the work, much of it will be familiar, but said in a new way and a way that will make a better story to tell your student as well. People with chronic pain generally no longer trust movement. Graded movement exposure is a non-harming way to rebuild that essential, embodied "home" for the student.

Sensation Lava Lamp: List your discomforts right now, choose one, watch it and the cascade of stimuli and the shape of the spaces or locations as they ebb, increase, flow, and shift. If my age is telling, search a video online if you don't know what a lava lamp is, as the visual is a great metaphor for the impermanent nature of outputs from our nervous system, to include pain. For people with chronic pain, it is counterintuitive that attending to sensation actually lessens discomfort, so start with a minor sensation not directly involved in *the* pain. After some success in noting change, then invite inquiry of the same nature around that bigger pain. Small doses (2–3 mins) a few times per day are a great start. For we professionals, dive right into your biggest, ugliest discomfort. Nothing to fear here.

Resistance is Futile: Practice noticing how often, and usually unconsciously, you want things to be different than the way they are. Notice when you want things you like to stay the way they are forever and what you do not like you want to disappear immediately. This is, of course, violence against self. Through the practice of living with things as they are, you will discover that, while life may not be less painful, your experience of it is substantially better. By fully accepting what is true in the moment we create the only firm place to begin to make changes in life. Want it to be otherwise? Caught ya!

Behold Beauty: Can you keep in the contours of your mind some small bit of beauty, even in your darkest times? Surely there's room for just a bit of beauty (nature, person, art, melody, etc.) not to rid the darkness, but, as O'Donohue (2017) suggests, "endure the bleakness." He noted that beauty is not a luxury, but what ennobles the heart and reminds us of the infinity that is within us. Holding a space for beauty reminds us of the presence of good that is so intimate and deep within us always. There's always room for just a bit of beauty too. What will your bit of beauty be today? Glance at it, hold it in your peripheral vision, and occasionally sustain it with your full attention.

Re-embodiment Practice: Disembodiment refers to the feeling of no longer having control over one's body, or not having ownership of one's body. Disembodiment metaphors are common and suggest that a person (me?) perceives that their body or body part no longer belongs to them, is unlikeable, or strange. Clues for noticing disembodiment range from direct statements such as "I can't find my hand" or "I've got a manikin leg," to more stealth ones such as "The knee's very tricky." Clue: The use of the, this, that, or it instead of my to refer to a part of the body suggests disembodiment. The exercise? Add "my" and state literally without metaphor what the experience(s) are for them (you) (Moseley and Butler 2017).

Not Enough? When feelings of inadequacy, vulnerability, longing, or not having enough arise and intrude into your awareness, pause. You cannot stop them from arising. But you assume control by changing how you perceive them. You can do that by refusing to identify with the feelings, stating they are neither you nor yours, then seeing them simply as transient emotional states of mind. Repetition is the key. Prevent the violence.

Threshold Drill: Pain and illness are just two forms of thresholds. We mentioned thresholds in the wisdom Time Thief practice. The root is "thresh" which means to separate the chaff from the grain, to get to what is essential. What happens if we begin to see these doorways that demand change and accept them as thresholds to step over into a new challenging, but critical and worthy, fullness for the transformations of us? What needs to be stripped, what will be left, and how bountiful might the yield be from the threshing? Try this framing and then consider more in the next exercise. Notice how many thresholds you literally step through during your day as well: in and out of your home, between rooms, entering businesses, places of worship. They are everywhere if we wake up to see.

Put a New Frame on It: Reframing is a powerful exercise and it doesn't require Freud's couch. Reframing includes altering the idea and/or emotional context or viewpoint relative to the situation in which it is experienced. The new "frame" is the changes made which ought to match the "facts" involved in the situation as well or better than the old frame. The new frame then changes the meaning, a part of identity as we've described earlier. First practice new frames on your own concepts or emotional setting. Sense what changes across all levels. Then begin to listen for situations others share and, when therapeutically appropriate, invite them to play with constructing new frames and sensing the associated changes. Yes, there is a relationship between this practice of frames and the lens swapping. Can you *see* the differences though, too?

Create New Social Settings: Try engaging in a new social setting where other people are counting on you. That new setting can alter the painful/uncomfortable consequences of novel atramovements which can be recontexualized as tolerable, even desirable, allowing you to tolerate more activity. A well-structured yoga class can be one example for students who can't think their way to that kind of pain tolerance, but being placed in a social situation like a class it is a likely outcome that can be helpful, given the principles of yoga for pain are adhered to in the class. When we change our social context, our drive as humans is so interested in one another that our social experiences utterly dominate our systems. Change your or their social experience, the brain changes focus and outputs.

Lizard Tanning: Many of the pain exercises available are centered on doing. That doing after all is the spirit of "can do" and excessive learned activism, but doing without a "why" as Meister Eckhart would say. Can you create experiences of deep solitude and silence, savoring the richness of the nothingness experience and of just doing nothing? In yoga we talk of calming the reptilian brain, since that brain is calmed by the lizard lying in the sun—doing nothing—just being, but in safety. This meets what Fox (2016, p.249) reported as the, "profound need of our time, to develop the mindfulness that can combat the excessive reptilian brain power trips that so dominate a patriarchal and imperial culture in its last days." The frequency prescription is daily, the duration dosage can be a small as five minutes. No sunscreen needed. Just "tan" peacefully, little lizard, you and your students.

Goldilocks Integration: Not too hot, not too small, just right. Sense your current emotional state. Positive emotions, like joy, love, awe, and happiness, can be considered increases in your level of integration. That's why they feel good. Negative emotions, such as anger, sadness, fear, disgust, and shame, might be considered as decreases in integration. And they feel bad. Siegel states that when such negative emotions are prolonged and intense, one can become prone to states of rigidity or chaos as integration is lowered over longer periods of time (2017, p.114). This exercise is when you sense positive emotions, can you identify the linkages present in your experience? Conversely, when you experience negative emotions, can you identify what you experience as either chaotic or rigid, and then see if you can make some linkages in the chaos and generate some differentiation amongst the rigid? Does that shift your emotional state? Our emotional state is a constant flow, so you can check in anytime. If you are comfortable with gunas, revisit that section of the book and apply the many aspects of Ayurveda as well.

Ahimsâ (Non-Harming) to Self: More ahimsâ, that's why it is the first yama. Our daily thoughts and decisions can be moments of violence to self. The violence isn't the same as someone hitting you or being abusive. Yet these same painful sensory experiences arise in reaction to our own thoughts or actions, and we fail to recognize our behavior as violent. Review the past 2–3 hours and see if you can recall this being the case. What will you do differently when you sense this next time? Ahimsâ rocks.

Time Out! Another clock practice. Abusing your time commitments is participating in violence against self. This may be in the form of overscheduling to the point that you are never still. Or it may be by allocating your time in a manner that doesn't reflect your inner priorities.

Both create strain and turbulence. We aren't machines designed to run at maximum capacity. Try making a list of your values and prioritize them, then compare those priorities with how you actually spend your time. Keep this list and check it each week as you plan your time. Schedule just "being" time and honor that as a high priority. Set the intention, set the schedule for a human, then review. Every week.

Creativity Practices

These practices offer primers as described in Chapter 5.

New Understandings about Creativity for You: Describe how your relationship with the concepts of creativity has changed, if it has, after reading and reflecting on that chapter.

Your Historical Creativity Reflection: Reflect on times you have felt "creative" in your yoga practice as a student, as a professional, as a yoga trainer of other professionals, or co-worker/partner in your yoga-related business. Have you continued to practice that behavior? Did it change the way you behaved in other circumstances? How could it have been even better? Give yourself the gift of the time to write out your answers versus "thinking them"…the psychomotor activity of writing is much more powerful. Then harvest future creative experiences the same way. Savor and delight.

Pay Attention!

> "Choice of attention—to pay attention to this or ignore that—is to the inner life what choice is to the outer life."
>
> W. H. Auden (1907–1973)

Attention Drill: Often, simplest is best. Focused attention is often people's first introduction to meditation/yoga. During focused attention, you learn to develop cognitive (thinking) control and attentional stability by sustaining focus on the moment-to-moment arising of sensory, emotional, and cognitive events. In doing so you attend to the dynamic nature of some chosen object of focus, most often the sensations of breath or body. When your attention drifts to a distracting sensory event, you note the distraction, smile softly, and disengage by returning your attention back to the object of focus. Over and over. The progression of difficulty is starting with breath, then emotions, and finally thoughts as focal points. Start with short sessions of a few minutes and build steadily.

Mindful Walking: We yoga professionals seem to be as busy as everyone else. Can you pay careful attention for even a short walk? Prove it. Let your entire body soften and receive the sounds, scents, touches, sights, and changing sensations. Gently watch how your thoughts and breathing respond, notice your self-congratulations, and come back to paying attention. Over and over and over. Returning to attention is victory. Walk the talk.

Noticing: Just begin to notice. Notice (pause momentarily) and ask, how did that happen? When a solution to a vexing problem comes to you. When you avoid an argument or resolve a conflict. When you utilize one of your favorite gadgets. When a student asks a question or makes a statement and you suddenly know what to do next (intuitive wisdom?). Or when you don't know what to do next. When you find yourself wasting time with TV or the internet. Over and over, just notice and ask silently, "What is happening now?" The acts of paying attention, pausing, and reflecting are of course the bedrock of clinical and professional mastery. I'm suggesting you merely redouble your practice of looking and asking, putting a novel demand on your nervous system to consider and filter in a way that is just a bit different than your habit. Noticing your noticing is critical behavior to move toward more experiences of ordinary and extraordinary creativity. You are on notice.

Sit Still: Can you? Not just your bones being still. How about your focus of attention? It is of course the nature of the mind to flit from point to point. Can you gently reign that attention to one point for a few breaths? For ten minutes daily observe your breathing pattern, noticing when you get distracted from paying attention and return to the task of paying attention with a gentle smile. The repetition strengthens your ability to attend, and with that to be present for creative new possibles. No attention, very few possibles.

Friendship Garden Exercise: In our hectic world, we've lost the art of growing friendships of depth. Deep social connection has big implications for relief of suffering and pain, but can't be left to chance. Pick one friend or someone you would like to be a friend. Think of your relationship as a new garden. What are the ingredients you will need? Can you afford to neglect the garden? How will it change? What surprises might there be? How long are you dedicated to cultivating whatever blooms and will you get around to weeding? One friendship for three months. Lucky friend. A great garden requires extended attention, but brings joy, beauty, and surprises.

Back to Here: There's a Tibetan saying, "Dwelling on the past brings remorseful thoughts and clinging to future increases our hopes and fears so let go of it" (Yanconpa (1213–1258), in Jinpa 2015, p.47). Develop the exercise of noticing when you have remorseful thoughts or are hoping or fearful, and then let go and ground back into sensing the present. Over and over, with a soft smile on each time you return to the present. How does that smile feel? How does your face change in the present versus the future or past? Use that as a reward for an exercise well done.

Submerse Your Attention into an Art Form: Find a piece of art or natural artifact. Can you allow yourself to fall deeply into that form and lose track of time and surroundings? Try this on a regular basis. You don't have to be "good" at it. It is just for your engagement and to redirect your attention from that smoking treadmill of thinking and doing behind your eyebrows. You will be making some buff attention muscles diving into the object and, most importantly, when you notice you've been distracted and return your attention. Just like the negative work of lifting weights. Slow and controlled.

Feelings... Way More Than Feelings

Breath: Emotions Link: Attending to our affect allows us to have space to respond rather than react to our environment (internal and external). Explore your breathing and watch your emotional state shift or alter your emotional state and watch your breath change. You know the drill: Breathe short and fast; now try one long sigh; how about holding your breath? Try on some more patterns and sense what happens to you emotionally. Then notice what your breath does when you act scared, happy, sexy, funny, curious, serious...keep going, what else changes? Pay attention to what happens with friends, students, at work, and so on.

It's literally everywhere and the more your exercise your intention to pay attention to feelings, well, just watch.

Range of Emotions: Our emotions affect learning, to include motor learning (asana) and pain perception/output, as we've explored. Sharpen your play with basic mindful emotional awareness exercises. Sit slumped, what emotion is that? Sit tall and straight, what is that? Celebrate, what is that? Anger? Show me by your posture. Thoughts are movements. Change the thoughts, movement changes…ask any elite athlete or performing artist. By the same token, posture influences mood and mood is affected by posture. How many emotions can you experience? Then start to notice how many you have every day. Each asana has an effect, or, said another way, is an expression of an emotional state. Notice them and share with your students.

Answer "How Are You?" Truthfully: Of course, only when it is socially and professionally appropriate. Or for fun, sometimes when it isn't! See what happens. Again, when it's appropriate, challenge someone to answer more fully when you inquire into their affective state and you get a rote reply. See if you can sense what they report. Practicing within and between sharpens our affective skill and maximizes the number of new possibles that can emerge at any time. Remember, oneself is a biggie in the wisdom formula. Wisdom = (Deep + Accurate Insights) x (Oneself + Central Existential Life Issues) + Skillful Benevolent Responsiveness.

Who Is in Charge Here? List your many relationships, both personal and professional, and then rank them along a spectrum of whether they feel like a partnership or whether someone is overly in charge/dominating the relationship. How about your relationship with yourself for various aspects of your life? Everybody getting along in there and working together? You and any loved ones? Between you and your students? Now journal what those relationships each feel like and how those feelings might shift if you changed the dynamic along the continuum. Affective sensitivity can allow us to know when creativity is threatened by a relationship out of balance. Looking is measuring and creates new possibles. Look, don't guess.

Boredom as Teacher: When you experience boredom either socially or professionally, note your posture/breath when you feel bored. Alter one or both and note what happens. What does boredom signal about your feelings? Your intention? Where was your attention when you discovered the boredom? Might boredom be an opposite of creativity or a spark for it? I'm betting boredom is a signal there is both depth and accuracy missing in the moment (minimal wisdom). Act to create a new possible after you welcome the perception.

What Are You Ingesting Emotionally? Pay more attention to what emotions the media you consume during the day creates in you. Be selective and make sure the diet nurtures rather than depletes you. The industries have invested heavily to excite and titillate you: Quite probably not in your best interest, or actually adding to your stress load, dampening the fostering of creative future actions by creating a less than optimal state. Also, pay attention to what your closest associates are serving as well. If need be, offer something more nourishing in response to less than emotionally nutritious sharing. Both are sound and visual "feeds" do just that: Feed us. Bon appetit.

The Best Intentions

Beauty Added to Your Usual Spaces Is a Spark: Is the beauty in your primary workspace limited to that tired old bamboo shoot or corn plant? Note how you shift when you introduce small things of beauty to your spaces. When did you stop noticing beauty was absent? What happens when you bring something new? What type of things are acceptable as beauty? Says who? Beauty isn't necessarily more of course, but do be deliberate in your intention to celebrate simple beauty and invite your students to the same practice. Keep it simple. Gazing upon the palm of your hand is hard to beat. Just stopping to notice can allow beauty to arise out of the ordinary and familiar.

Create a "Between" Students or Classes Mindful Ritual: Do you have a practice of grounding and presence when you transition between students or classes? How about at other times during the day? Setting or resetting intention activates your nervous system to stay aware of related sensory input that will support your intention. But, like our electronics, going too long without rebooting allows systems to get overloaded and those inputs that might spark a creative moment get lost in the slow, overwhelmed systems of sensory information. Saying a prayer/setting an intention for the former or next activity while sensing yourself provides that important reboot on the run. Exhale more deeply three times while sensing the support of the floor beneath you, let the creativity emerge in line with your intention.

Metta (Kindness) Meditation Practice: Many of you will know this practice. It is Buddhist in origin, but non-denominational to fit with any traditional spiritual practice. Your intention of holding yourself, loved ones, and others in your heart and wishing them well is a repeated intentional practice. Sensing those you are focusing on in your heart space makes for an embodied primer of creativity as well. One script: May all beings attain happiness and its causes. May all beings be free from suffering and its causes. May all beings never be separated from joy that is free of misery. May all beings abide in equanimity, free from bias of attachment and aversion (Jinpa 2015).

Explore Nonviolent Communication Practices: Language reveals our thoughts and activates action. Gaining enhanced insight into how language drives intention is invaluable. Explore the writings and practices of the late Marshall B. Rosenberg's organization, many of which are free (Rosenberg 2005). Ahimsâ (non-harming) is our first yama. Modifying our language toward that purpose will create less harming. They also share an amazing list of words to expand our choices in communicating our emotions and needs. More possibles, more actuals.

Prayer Practices: The tonglen practice, rosary, mala bead practice, and morning/evening prayer are all tried and true practices. They are great techniques for generating enhanced intentional awareness. They prime us for the day ahead and celebrate the day behind us. The refocusing of attention to intention fires patterns to refresh and promote integration while reinforcing our innate tendency to prosocial behavior. My dear spiritual mentor, Fr. Mike Librandi, finished every one of his brief, brilliant sermons with, "Think about it, pray about it."

Engaging: Moving into New Territories

Increase Your Use of Metaphor and Images: In your personal and professional practices, intentionally increase your use of both metaphor and images to an almost uncomfortable level for you. Note how the others respond and seek their feedback. You can also jot down new favorite metaphors from classes you attend or those you find while reading or conversing. Make it your new collection. As you teach, learn from your students by asking them to share their experiences using metaphors they create or the two of you discover together. They are lurking everywhere. Why that was one in the last sentence. And another.

Contemplative Prophet/Profit: You can't put those two synonyms together! I did. As yoga professionals by an expanded definition, we must confront the importance of our prophetic as distinct from our contemplative vocation. We must be both, and our creativity does not stand apart from our values and priorities. So, as you do your business planning and lay out your strategies, can you also contemplate how those plans (profit) reflect your responsibility as a yoga professional to be a change agent in your community (prophet)? It isn't an either/or question, it's a both. Every business decision as you engage your new yoga. The profitable prophet: You create how you will *actually* show up.

Practice the Better: Rohr (2011) stated one of the guiding principles of his Center for Action and Contemplation is that the best criticism of the bad is the practice of the better. When you encounter something you automatically label "bad" during your day, pause and see if you can identify what the "better" is and engage in that better. Bad signals better. You will be busy.

Working It: Seeing this world of creative connection in work relationships can be an opportunity to connect and create. Are we seeking to control others, to box them in, to have them conform to the picture we have decided we want to see, or are we allowing them to speak, to be who they are; are we open to experience them? Do we know how to listen in a way that allows their creativity and ours to flourish? Are we seeing and hearing them? Are we making a space for them to emerge along with us? Do we know how to look, to listen, to encourage, to play, to engage with others in a way that allows our creativities to connect, so that we may create together? If we ever doubt that we are able to answer these questions, we can draw inspiration from these two remarks. The first is from Martin Luther King: "Our true nature is creativity" (cited in Fox

2004b, p.28). Whether we call it an "unconscious process, an impersonal Brahman, or a Personal Being of matchless power and infinite love, there is a creative force in this universe that works to bring the disconnected aspects of reality into a harmonious whole" (Fox 2004b, p.58). Engage in harmonious work creation.

Do the Raisin Mindfulness Exercise: If you haven't yet tried this classic practice made famous by Jon Kabat Zinn, find it online. It is easy to do. If you don't like raisins, a piece of chocolate works too. We used to have wrapped chocolates with the exercise description posted next to the bowl in our clinic. Most people just gobbled the candy mindlessly though! After you complete the exercise, try to make it a practice for at least one mouthful of food a meal. What else are you chewing on that would benefit from adopting this practice?

Try a New Mindbody Practice: Aikido, tai chi, dance, martial arts, pottery, tumbling, acrobatics, acupuncture, anything that will be a new experience. Observe and sense all your responses and reactions from a new student's perspective. This experience will enhance your empathy for what by now is a distant memory of how it was when you first stepped on the mat. Be sure the new practice has your interest and is novel. That neuroplastics thing.

Teach Breath Awareness Anew Again: This follows the old teaching adage of engagement along the lines of watch one, do one, teach one vein. Try it with a favorite, comfortable student and get their feedback/contribution as you describe what you see and have them describe what they experience in sensing their breath. The vayus make a great beginning graphic for each of you to consider as you create your report of what you can and can't feel. Then find times to insert it into the day at traffic lights, on hold, in line, or as you settle into bed. See if you can recall and employ that wide-eyed wonder of the novice each time, trying to glimpse where the breath emerges from and where it retreats to each breath. The practice never gets old, but employs all of Halifax's (2012) domains for compassion and therefore creativity priming.

Seeing Into...In-Sights

Book Diet: They call them sacred texts for a reason. Some classical, some more esoteric, but those containing writings of sages and mystics. Think of them as the power smoothies of your reading diet in contrast to the junk food soundbites we take in most days. Going back to the primary sources of your yoga and spiritual practices is steeped in nutrition for us. Carve out time each day to refresh and nourish yourself. This can be fodder for your contemplation exercise described elsewhere. A real two-for-one and no calories.

Explore across the Disciplines: At least once a month take an hour or so to read a few short pieces from disciplines or perspectives that are very different from yours. Discover what you see through the new lens. What's your bodily, breath, or emotional response to the work? Any insights pertinent to your "world"? Are your students bound in a limited, self-reinforcing diet of information and perspectives as well? Break down what we now call the "echo" of media.

Beauty or Glamour? O'Donohue (2017) asserted that as a culture we have lost the ability to discern between beauty and glamour, often mistakenly chasing the latter. How do you define beauty? How is it different than glamour? When things either strongly attract or repulse you, pause and consider what is triggering that response in you? Can there be beauty in the "negative," such as death, illness, trauma? Can there be wrong action in what is glamorous or popular, underpinned by wrong action? Discerning the source of your desires and looking deeply will lead to many new insights and the relief of future suffering. Something as routine as hair coloring or teeth whitening, when held in steady awareness, can generate new and possibly more accurate insights à la wisdom.

Study and Practice the Insight Meditation Techniques: These you know from your yoga training. Are they part of your current practice? What's been your experience with them? When's the last time you modified your meditation practice? Why or why not? A slight tweak might crack open whole new insights. You can always return to the familiar. Bring along your body and engage. They are not thought exercises.

Check Out Contemplative Practices: All major religions have them. The famous Trappist monk, Thomas Merton, said of contemplation, "It is spiritual wonder. It is spontaneous awe at the sacredness of life, of being. It is gratitude for life, for awareness and for being" (cited in Fox 2016, p.47). Try one that matches your interests and see if there is a local group that practices. They are not the same as some of the classic yoga practices, so, if you aren't familiar, spice up your practice with one that draws your attention.

Modern Self-Study (Svadhyaya): There are numerous online tests such as Enneagram, Myers-Briggs, Disc personality inventory, and so on. They can be rabbit holes too, so sample, note what you discover, and use what works for you. Then see if you can find the yoga equivalent. In addition to offering you insights, this can be familiar "Western" language to bridge your student's understanding with older traditions in yoga. You can also engage mental health professionals because of the familiarity, but introduce how these limbs affect the physical and pain outputs, thoughtfully leaving the mental domain to them. You need to know *you* to tip-toe along that conversation. *Oneself* comes first in defining wisdom after all.

"Yes, and": Practice answering all questions with the non-dual expression of Richard Rohr's (2013) book title, *Yes, and…* The discipline of having to acknowledge others' statements and complete your assertions and answers with "Yes, and…" is clumsy at first, but I promise there'll be a bonanza of insights awaiting you as unearth the hard-packed habit of giving the "right" answer. You can also practice internally as you self-reflect on your conversations as move through your day. When you sense you just arrived at an answer, insert the "Yes, and…" to gain further insight.

Enhance or Start a Mentor:Mentee Relationship: Be both a mentor and a mentee. If you are already one of each, freshen up the relationship by sharing what you are discovering here in this book. If you are "guru-shy," study the difference between a healthy mentoring relationship and a traditional guru relationship. Both can be powerful in the right circumstances, but either can slip into an unhealthy relationship without sufficient awareness and communication. I have found being a mentee beneficial for helping me to see what I couldn't see either by habit or inexperience. As a mentor, I learn constantly from others while reaping the benefit of supporting another. The way it should be.

Embodying: Sensing Calls from Inside

Contraction or Expansion? Sharon Salzberg (2017) wrote a fascinating blog post about the literal embodied experience of contracting versus expanding. The gist shared the neuroscience of what we literally sense in our bodies happening when we are thinking inclusively as "us" (Siegel's mWe I suspect) is that one feels more expansive, while when we other, "us versus them," there's an embodied sense of shrinkage or contracting. I have practiced this and found it fascinating. Here's what you do. Next time you are in situation with dear friends feeling great, pause and sense how "big" you feel in the space. Then to experiment, make a judgment to yourself about someone you are with (that's a weird shirt, she ought to lose that guy, etc.) and recheck to sense your size. You can also play the same way with your students. If you are listening to them recount a pain challenge and note you are "seeing" their story as only their pain (them), check your size. Then gently see what happens to your shape as you allow that suffering to be yours as well. Did you change? Of course, you want to maintain your self-care to avoid vicarious trauma over time, but I suspect developing the ability to move back and forth, using your embodied awareness of your state of contraction/expansion will be a tool for both empathic presence and self-care.

Freshen Up Your Asana: I assume most of you have had a long-standing asana practice. When's the last time you really shook it up and made the routine new? Butera and Elgelid (2017) have a great resource for doing so. We know novelty of inputs is what drives change in the nervous system and prompts integration along with reorganization. They offer a full spectrum of strategies as well as in-depth scientific rationale for doing so. Try studying the meanings behind the names of asana and see if you can sense those meanings in your body. Add some somatic lessons between your rote expression of the asana and post-lesson. What did you notice? Can you transfer any of these new experiences into your daily movements? Each time you invite a new way of being in your body you disrupt (perturb) the deep patterns and invite new connections. Make the old new again.

Sex…Not as a Tantric Practice: Sex, of course, is the only reason we are all here. But like all behavior, without attention and cultivation, we can fall into habitual patterns. Eros is the basic life force and has a rich influence on yoga practices. If your sex life isn't nourishing and energizing, there are quality, highly trained and regulated professionals (counselors, physiotherapists, physicians, etc.) who can support your development of this critical part of being embodied. This is also a key component of life to inquire about for your students with chronic pain. Few people, if anyone, ever ask about their sex life. Just asking is a relief, and of course having resources to direct the person to for support can be a breakthrough for the person. Sex shouldn't hurt and there are resources available to express Eros despite pain. Sex definitely shouldn't be dull either. Celebrate Shiva and Shakti enfleshed in a culturally appropriate manner.

Play More: Ask yourself, "What do I play at?" And then ask your students. In my experience, "Not much or nothing" are the usual answers. We have all become so dreadfully serious. What does it feel like inside you during play? You may have to seek consultation from some three or four-year-olds if it's been a while. Can you schedule some play with the same sincerity you do all your other tasks, as well as being open to spontaneous opportunities that arise? Are the classes you attend or teach playful? If not, why not? Evolutionarily continuing to play through adulthood is what distinguishes we adult humans from our other primate relatives. Have you expressed that difference recently? No rules, make it fun, and no agenda other than to just *be* that little kid having fun with new crayons or a pile of empty boxes.

Savasana (Corpse) Exercise: There is a saying in the Tibetan tradition that the best measure of spiritual development is how one relates to death when that day arrives. We practice savasana pose in order to leave at the last breath, hopefully with a sense of joy, but at least with no remorse. Enhancing our awareness of our mortality helps us align our deepest aspirations with our everyday actions. Be warned it can also, according to Jinpa (2015), bring a kind of brutal honesty—and courage—to our life. Jennifer Taylor's (2008) article is full of appropriate ways to introduce end of life conversations and explorations into yoga therapy. The repeated practice leaves little room for false pretense or maintaining a façade, and reveals the fruitlessness of expending too much energy taking care of our small self. Die daily. You are anyway.

Bhavana/Guided Imagery: Could it be your bhavana practice has grown stale too? Luckily modern technology gives us so much access to new forms and teachers across many disciplines that use imagery. Develop an expanding library of resources, diving deeply in and sensing the shifts in your internal landscape as you do so. Reflect on your experience afterward and note if there might be a place for expanding such a practice in your own self-care or to use the material professionally with your students. Then as you teach and are leading an imagery, see if you can get out of your own way and allow the imagery to emerge from your own felt internal sense versus trying to repeat someone else's exact script from a different circumstance. This emergent property of creative new imageries is a source of constant surprise and amazement for me as I too get to hear them emerge from my own voice. I can see you doing it.

Practices Without a Home

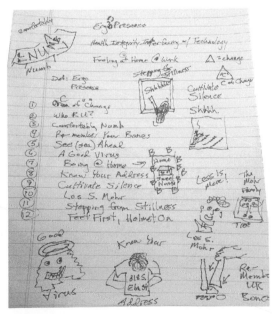

Word Play

Word Play: Capture word plays related to your work. Sketch out silly images that reinforce the principles you share. Invite students to create and share theirs, where you all learn from one another, uncovering metaphors and assumptions that might otherwise be missed or cause suffering left unaware. No drawing skills required. Here are a few of mine to get you started (see the figure above).

- ErgoPresence: Health Integrity Interfacing with Technology

- Feeling @ home @ work

- (Delta = change) C (sea) of Change

- Who R U?

- Comfortably Numb

- Re-member U-R bones

- See (sea) Ahead

- A Good Virus

- Being @ home

- Know Your Address

- Cultivate Silence

- Les S Mohr

- Stepping from Stillness

- Feet First, Helmet On

Simplify: Whenever you teach or are taught, simplify as best you can. To simplify is "When you reach a point where you have achieved transparency (laying bare the underlying truth whatever it reveals), clarity (expressing meaning clearly and simply), and usability (making something fit for its purpose), you have likely achieved simplicity" (Siegel and Etzkorn 2013, p.6). This skill of simplifying is exactly what makes for a good quote. Consider:

- "Making the simple complicated is commonplace; making the complicated simple…that's creativity." —Charles Mingus

- "More important than the quest for certainty is the quest for clarity." —François Gautier

- "You can't heal, won't you don't feel." —Unknown

- "Yoga is known through yoga." —Vyasa

- "Pain invites Wisdom forward." —Me, just now

- Simply fun to simplify.

How Do You Measure Up? We yoga professionals know how to teach from the whole person perspective, or at least that's what we claim. Good news, you don't have to guess whether you can or not, there's a study with a reliable scale to help you "see" just how integrated your time with your student is. The study (Van de Velde *et al.* 2016) and scale is free here: http://journals.plos.org/plosone/article?id=10.1371/journal.pone.0164018. When recording your answers, use your most recent student of private instruction. Let me know how you measure up.

The Power of Story: He must think storytelling is really important? Again? Yes, once more. A slightly different take in this practice to expand on how good storytelling changes our world. There is no power greater than a community discovering what it cares about, and this includes your teaching both individual and group classes. Ask "What's possible?" not "What's wrong?" Keep asking. Notice what you and they care about. Rather than hold back, assume that many others share your dreams. Be brave enough to start a conversation that matters. (Courage comes from the Old French word for heart: *cuer.*) Converse with people you know. Talk to people you don't know. Dialog with people you never talk to. Be intrigued by the differences you hear: Gregory Bateson's "differences that make a difference." Expect to be surprised and to surprise others. Can you value your curiosity more than certainty? Invite in everybody who cares to work on what's possible. From our story, earlier in this book, we know that creative solutions come from new connections. Keep in mind, we don't fear people whose story we know. Real listening always brings human beings closer together. Meaningful conversations can change our world. Exercise your power. Spin a better yarn.

Gratitude: Rohr (2011) stated, in effect, that our concern is not so much to have what we love anymore, but to love what we have right now. This gratitude practice is to pause, sense what you have in this moment, right now. Can you be grateful for whatever that is? Does that gratitude create an embodied sensation you can attend to? Can you sustain that gratitude for several breaths? Is there something else right now for which you can be grateful? Repeat and enjoy (bring in-joy).

Finding Right Work: Many of our students spend over one-third of their lives in the workplace. And one of the loneliest and most painful things you can find is somebody who is in the wrong kind of work, who shouldn't be doing what they are doing. Quite possibly they should be doing something else and haven't the courage to get up and leave it and make a new possibility for themselves. Certainly, there are many times people can't leave, but, in my experience, it often hasn't even been considered. Often their workplace is dedicated to productivity and looking at the bottom line only. While we are not vocational counselors by any means, right work is crucial and if our students stand back a little and discover in their practice that their spirit and soul dimensions are not luxury items, but are the very origins and sources of work which will enable everything to flow and unfold in a new way. If we can, then they (and we) realize that the invisible world is a secret, hidden resource that can be released and excavated for the huge resources of spirit, guidance, and for areas of themselves that they've forgotten. An exploration of Ayurveda can be fruitful here as well if that isn't familiar to you. Seems like right work for us.

Non-Grasping as a Business Plan: Fox (2016, p.137) stated, "A merchant mentality leads us down a false path of ownership, whereas in fact all in life is on a loan… Instead of grabbing, hoarding, possessing, clinging, Eckhart teaches letting go (Abgeschiedeneheit) and letting be (Gelassenheit)." Our yamas and niyamas are everywhere, to include this call for aparigraha and santosha from a German mystic long ago. Yes, and…you have to pay rent, eat, and those other realities of life. But as yoga professionals we must also consider are we "producing" to bring forward truth, belief, love, acceptance, fellowship, and understanding? Certainly, there are plenty of yogis selling abundance courses, but, if they make it sound simple, they're selling soulless materialism, not our new yoga. Where's the path for you? I don't know. Your circumstances are uniquely yours alone. As you work "on" your business though, brings these ethical practices front and center, every time.

Transformative Leadership: Regardless if you are just leading your own two feet into the bathroom in the morning or have 10,000 social media followers following your lead, our world needs a new kind of leader. Our era of uncertainty described in the creativity chapter demands a new form of leadership. My doctoral advisor and dissertation chairman, Dr. Alfonso Montuori, PhD, has studied and written about this topic extensively (Montuori and Donnelly in press). Transformative leadership proposes that everybody can lead and create, and in fact, does lead, even if only by example. Consistent with earlier chapters, a transformative leader acknowledges the larger context in our moment of global transformation, and recognizes the way all human beings participate in the future creation. The authors admonish that we are the transformation, and our choices and actions, our ways of being, relating, knowing, teaching, and doing, all contribute to the direction the transformation will take.

Transformative leadership involves embodying and taking responsibility for one's leadership and creativity. Montuori and Donnelly describe transformative leadership as "among other things, *a practice of unveiling our own creativity and leadership*, taking responsibility for them, and applying them to mutual benefit, creating collaboration and participatory leadership." Transformative leadership is an invitation to participate in a collective journey into the future, a journey of creative inquiry, creating ourselves, our relationships, and our communities as we've described in each of the preceding practices. Jinpa (2015, p.225) would add that compassion, personal integrity, humility, being open to others' perspectives yet taking responsibility to lead, all rooted in courage and a quiet confidence combine as the marks of truly great leaders. How do you lead? Do you lead? Think about it. Journal around the topics based on what you've read here. We all need your leadership, as well as that of your students.

Leaning in Business Asana: Just as in physical asana, where there is the temptation to lean on props or hang on our joints rather than execute right alignment, so too in our business dealings. "From now on Brother, everybody stands on his own feet." Thomas Merton commented: "We can no longer rely on being supported by structures that may be destroyed at any moment by a political power or a political force… The time for relying on structures has disappeared" (cited in Fox 2016, p.203). Merton was prophetically describing our current state where government, education, economics, and media are quaking under unsustainable stressors. As you create, beware of "leaning" on old, tired models. Seek new ways and dare to be the first. Review your business structure and note where you are leaning. Then make the postural corrections your business needs now.

A Pause

Avoid the temptation to allow these many practices to create a sense of overwhelm. Remember this teaching from wisdom is an ongoing, unfolding process, not an event. There is no endpoint to arrive at on time. Rather, think of these practices and the ones ahead as new friends with which to develop a relationship over time. Some you will visit often, others maybe only once or occasionally. With others you may decide to break off the friendship. That's what we discuss next. How and when to say "goodbye."

When to Change Practices

A common question that arises as people begin this creative process is "How do I know I'm on the right path?" and the related question "When should I change my practice?" The vexing thing about this embracing uncertainty stuff is quite often the answer is "It depends." Not very satisfying, is it? There are some pretty obvious answers. If what you are doing is generating greater pain and suffering for you or your students beyond just the modest discomfort of change, then by all means reassess, change the practice, and monitor the results, as with any yoga practice. I am also assuming that as a yoga professional you know the contraindications for the various yoga technologies and are modifying the practices accordingly. We won't be addressing those as the contraindications are readily available and should have been part of your training. If they weren't, study is ahead for you.

Now the less obvious answers. For instance, you've been doing such and such a practice for X number of weeks and nothing has changed, when do you change your practice? You don't want to be impatient and flitting from one practice to the next without allowing sufficient time, but you also don't want to be wasting time and resources on some practice that does not appear to be having any effect. My apologies in advance, but this discerning the difference of course is part of being a professional versus a technician. If I had your answers, you would just be a technician. Allow me to offer a checklist framework for review, but ultimately the decision will be yours for your practice, and the student's in consultation with you, for their practice. To paraphrase what is often attributed to Thomas Edison as he created the light bulb, "Well now we know what doesn't work." So, before you change course on these gray area assessments of practice effectiveness, consider the following:

1. What was the intention behind starting the practice? Have you maintained the intention or was it misguided upon reflection?

2. Was there anything you/your student discovered to date of value or benefit? If so, might more be in the offing?

3. Has this practice illuminated some other insight that suggests a new possible you/they would like to explore instead? If so, would you continue this practice and add the new one or just replace the practice? And why?

4. Would there be any harm or cost to dropping this practice? How does that balance with any perceived benefit? Basic cost/benefit analysis.

5. Have you or your student consulted with your local community or sangha for additional perspectives or insight? Remember the individual is limited and having others' inputs can reveal blind spots in our assessment.

6. Have you returned to one or more of the making space practices with the intention of seeking direction around this practice in question? If not, you know what to do.

7. You can always return to the practice if you miss it, or drop it in the future if you intend to continue at this point, so decide, and act now.

Be on the alert for boredom, routine, mind-wandering, and avoidance as the symptoms that should point you back to reviewing the above list. The freedom of the creative response allows us the privilege to crumple up another page, or break the clay pot, and start over. From before we first successfully negotiated our little chubby fist into our mouth as an infant, life has been a series of explorations and testing. Sustaining presence as best we can and avoiding violence as the only real constraints. You and your student now have the power and are the wisdom, so go!

Let's head to the woods a moment before we finish…

MINNESOTA ADVENTURE

Had someone told me even a part of what was to become of my life and work back then as I lay staring at the ceiling in that Minnesota cabin, I couldn't have laughed at them because that would have hurt too much. I'd probably have just cussed a bit of a blue streak and suggested our visit was over because they were talking nonsense and I was in no mood for pipe dreams. At that time, I was still very much entrapped by my family of origin and cultural list of possibles. I could only see what I knew. And I know, in my quest for certainty and limited possibles, I would have dispelled the suggestion of such new possibles, and what are now, indeed, my actuals, as ridiculous. I was unaware of my inherent creative nature, the power of suffering to transform one's self-definition, and as such, one's role or dharma in the world. Me, a conservative, military-trained, "objective" healthcare professional writing a book for yoga professionals for a United Kingdom publisher... right! And yet that is my current actual, and each key stroke generates more actuals, and from them new possibles for me as the author, but ultimately for you the reader and your students. I can't wait for the next surprise, so let's head to a brief concluding chapter and get you set with your new possibles to ease the present and future suffering in our world! We are transformative leaders.

· · ·

A Special Bonus for Making It to the End!

Oh, alright, and here's your recipe for your creative response through yoga therapy by teaching from the wisdom of pain. I couldn't leave us hanging without a "recipe":

Recipe

This recipe shall be known as: *Teaching from the Wisdom of Pain*

From the kitchen of: *Matt "Matman" Taylor*   This recipe serves: *Everyone*

Ingredients

Humility
Sense of Playfulness
Wisdom Practiced
Presence
Regular Practice
Primed for Creativity
Pain Literate
Sense of Humor

Directions

Practice the new yoga daily. Mix in plenty of playfulness and a big dose of humor, taking neither you or the suffering too seriously. Stay current on modern pain theory; remain primed to express your innate creativity with the students' creativity. Baked under the watchful eye of Presence, season with the wisdom you are, and remember, it isn't you doing the work Arjuna. Let rest and serve big portions! Enjoy.

Conclusion

You've made it to the end of the book. Thank you for staying with the process. I'm wondering what your experience has been? We have covered a great deal of material and unearthed more questions than answers. Has that been unsettling or, strangely, did it bring an ease to an unsettled experience that was there before we started? As with any wisdom exploration, chances are that "both/and" is the answer to that question. I know it is for me. I am both more unsettled in any sense of certainty, but breathing and moving from a deeper place of settled stillness. Fr. Rohr and Mary Catherine Bateson's use of the metaphor "home" that we explored in Chapter 3 on wisdom seems fitting. Home is not a place to retreat to away from Life, but it's that place from which we move out into the world to fully participate in creating and working to relieve present and future suffering for ourselves and others.

Conventional publishing wants me to make you feel safe and confident (at home) so you put this book down feeling assured and confident. It is in this part of the book where I am to write my "proof of thesis." In other words, tell you what I told you was right. Can you now see how even this long-standing feature of publishing is our collective, tired quest for certainty? We began the book asking why there are so many books and other resources on pain, and yet the problem of pain is skyrocketing? Right now, I'm wondering if I just added to that pile without any effect? If I could just "prove" what I have shared is the solution, then you and I could both rest easy knowing we were on the right path. Home sweet home.

But, alas, probably the best I can hope for is that being equipped now with some new perspectives and practices, I have primed you and those you interact with for the best chance of generating new possibles that enable more flourishing of new actuals in the future. What that future will look like no one knows. And that's OK. We do the practices, we let loose Arjuna's arrow of possible actions in this moment, and surrender the result of the new actual to Ishvara in whatever way we relate to that larger-than-us concept of creation. And repeat. Carrying ahimsā (non-harming) as our highest standard and intention in selecting from the new possibles, and then acting from the steadiness and equipoise in the asana of implementation. So simple and so hard.

This conclusion has no new assignment beyond what we've already covered. If there's one "exercise," it would be to share your feedback with me. If I have a reputation on any level, it would be that I am responsive to personal inquiries. I would love to learn about your experience while reading this book and exploring the practices. I will sustain my reputation, and personally respond to any inquiries you make to my attention. Each of us is so privileged to be in this constant flow of action: feedback: reflection: action. The sacred dance we described in the wisdom chapter. My receiving feedback from you and responding is as close as I will get to dancing and still have your toes safely protected from my two big left feet! I look forward learning from and with you, as we breathe together to birth forward our best possible future.

As we began, we finish. Back in the cabin in northern Minnesota…

MINNESOTA TIE-IN

Darkness has descended. The campfires and conversations around fire pits are silenced. The cabin is quiet, save the soft breathing of my wife lying gingerly alongside me on our snug little double bed. She's trying her best to not to jostle me. The window is open, trusting the screen to keep the horde of mosquitoes at bay on the other side. I had dozed off and on all day, and now sleep won't come.

Amid the night stillness, tucked among my worries and fears, a deep quieting settles in throughout the lakeside cabins. What's next? How am I going to be OK? Will my family be OK? I must be able to work and I am self-employed, so no disability safety net. And on and on… But somewhere, penetrating the noise of my fears, there emerges out of the surrounding darkness and the silence of nature, behind the chorus of crickets and cicadas, a haunting call of a loon for me to experience. Silence follows, but then, from somewhere deeper in the silence, another loon returns the call. And a new possible emerges from the ongoing groans of creation as I surrender to not knowing, but knowing I am home in some unexplainable way.

May you and those you serve find similar rest and ease as our future unfolds with so many new possibles for our collective home.

Thank you.

References

Allen, D. (2002) *Getting Things Done: The Art of Stress-Free Productivity.* New York: Penguin.

Aurobindo, S. (1993) *Integral Yoga: Sri Aurobindo's Teaching & Method of Practice.* Pondicherry, India: Sri Aurobindo Ashram Trust.

Bhagavad Gita 2:47 Accessed January 18, 2018 at www.holy-bhagavad-gita.org/chapter/2/verse/47.

Barron, F. (1990) *No Rootless Flower: Towards an Ecology of Creativity.* Cresskill, NJ: Hampton Press.

Bateson, G. (2000) *Steps to an Ecology of Mind.* Chicago, IL: University of Chicago Press.

Bateson, M. C. (2017) "Composing a Life." Interview with Krista Tippett, August 3. Accessed January 18, 2018 at https://onbeing.org/programs/mary-catherine-bateson-composing-a-life-aug2017.

Bateson, N. (2017) *Small Arcs of Larger Circles: Framing through Other Patterns.* Axminster: Triarchy Press.

Bocchi, G. and Ceruti, M. (2002) *The Narrative Universe.* Cresskill, NJ: Hampton Press.

Bruner, J. (1997) *On Knowing: Essays for the Left Hand,* 2nd edn. Boston, MA: Belknap Press.

Butera, K. and Elgelid, S. (2017) *Yoga Therapy: A Personalized Approach for Your Active Lifestyle.* Champaign, IL: Human Kinetics.

Capra, F. and Luisi, P. L. (2016) *The Systems View of Life: A Unifying Vision.* Cambridge: Cambridge University Press.

Cooper, D. (1990) *Existentialism.* Oxford: Blackwell.

Craig, A. D. (2015) *How Do You Feel?* Princeton, NJ: Princeton University Press.

Crisfield, L. (2017) "Why Yoga Is Not the Stilling of the Fluctuations of the Mind." Accessed January 18, 2018 at www.lucycrisfield.com/list-of-articles/why-yoga-is-not-the-stilling-of-the-fluctuations-of-the-mind.

Feuerstein, G. (1998) *The Yoga Tradition.* Prescott, AZ: Hohm Press.

Feuerstein, G. (2014) "Wisdom: The Hindu Experience and Perspective." In R. Walsh (ed.) *The World's Great Wisdom*. Albany, NY: SUNY Press.

Fox, M. (2004a) *One River, Many Wells: Wisdom Springing from Global Faiths*. New York: Penguin.

Fox, M. (2004b) *Creativity: Where the Divine and the Human Meet*. New York: Penguin.

Fox, M. (2016) *A Way to God: Thomas Merton's Creation Spirituality Journey*. Novato, CA: New World Library.

Garchar, K. (2012) "Imperfection, practice and humility in clinical ethics." *Journal of Evaluation in Clinical Practice 18*, 5, 1365–2753.

Gates, J. (2006) *Yogini: The Power of Women in Yoga*. San Rafael, CA: Mandhala Books.

Ghose, P. (ed.) (2016) *Einstein, Tagore and the Nature of Reality*. New York: Routledge.

Gilbert, P., Catarino, F., Duarte, C., Matos, M., *et al.* (2017) "The development of compassionate engagement and action scales for self and others." *Journal of Compassionate Health Care 4*, 4.

Gilbert, P., McEwan, K., Matos, M., and Rivis, A. (2011) "Fears of compassion: Development of three self-reported measures." *British Psychological Society 84*, 239–255. Scale accessed January 18, 2018 at https://compassionatemind.co.uk/uploads/files/fears-of-compassion-scale.pdf.

Gottschal, J. (2012) *The Storytelling Animal: How Stories Make Us Human*. New York: Houghton Mifflin Harcourt.

Govindarajan, V. and Trimble, C. (2013) *Beyond the Idea*. New York: St. Martin's Press.

Halifax, J. (2012) "A heuristic model of enactive compassion." *Current Opinion in Supportive and Palliative Care 6*, 2, 228–235.

Haskell, D. G. (2017) *The Songs of Trees: Stories from Nature's Great Connectors*. New York: Viking Press.

Heisenberg, W. (1958) *Physics and Philosophy: The Revolution in Modern Science*. New York: Prometheus Books.

Horton, C. A. (2012) *Yoga PH.D.* Chicago: Kleio Books.

Huxley, A. (2004) *The Perennial Philosophy*. New York: Harper Perennial.

Jinpa, T. (2015) *A Fearless Heart*. New York: Hudson Street Press.

Jung, C. G. (1980) *The Collected Works of C. G. Jung, Volume 1, Psychiatric Studies*. Princeton, NJ: Princeton University Press.

Kauffman, S. A. (2016) *Humanity in a Creative Universe*. New York: Oxford University Press.

Kelley, T. and Kelley, D. (2013) *Creative Confidence*. New York: Crown Publishing.

Khalsa, S. B. (2017) "The Road to Incorporating Yoga Therapy into Healthcare." Plenary address, Symposium on Yoga Therapy and Research (SYTAR), Newport Beach, CA.

King, M. L. (1958) *Stride toward Freedom: The Montgomery Story*. New York: Ballantine.

Kleim, J. (2015) "Neuroplasticity in Rehabilitation." Notes from lecture, Arizona PT Directors Meeting, Fall, Gateway Community College, Phoenix, AZ.

Kleim, J. and Jones, T. (2008) 'Principles of experience-dependent neural plasticity: Implications for rehabilitation after brain damage.' *Journal of Speech, Language, and Hearing Research 51*, Feb., S225–S239.

Mallinson, J. and Singleton, M. (2017) *Roots of Yoga*. New York: Penguin Classics.

Montuori, A. (2011) "Systems Approach." In M. Runco and S. Pritzker (eds.) *The Encyclopedia of Creativity* 2. San Diego, CA: Academic Press.

Montuori, A. (2017) "The evolution of creativity." *Collective Enlightenment, Spanda Journal* 7, 1, 147–156.

Montuori, A and Donnelly, G. (in press) "Transformative Leadership." In J. Neal (ed.) *The Handbook of Personal and Organizational Transformation.* New York: Springer.

Montuori, A. and Purser, R. (1997) 'Le dimensioni sociali della creatività.' *Pluriverso 1*, 2, 78–88.

Moseley, L. and Butler, D. (2017) *Explain Pain Supercharged.* Adelaide, Australia: Noigroup Publications.

Neff, K. (2011) *Self-Compassion: The Proven Power of Being Kind to Yourself.* New York: Harper Collins.

Nichol, L. (ed.) (2006) *David Bohm on Creativity.* New York: Routledge.

O'Donohue, J. (2017) "The Inner Landscape of Beauty." Accessed on January 18, 2018 at https://onbeing.org/programs/john-odonohue-the-inner-landscape-of-beauty-aug2017.

O'Mahony, S. (2017) "Compassion, Empathy, Flapdoodle." Accessed September 23, 2017 at http://www.drb.ie/essays/compassion-empathy-flapdoodle.

Ortner, C. N. M., Kilner, S. J., and Zelazo, P. D. (2007) 'Mindfulness meditation and reduced emotional interference on a cognitive task.' *Motivation Emotion 31*, 271–283.

Parameshwaran, D. and Thiagarajan, T. C. (2017) "Modernization, Wealth and the Emergence of Strong Alpha Oscillations in the Human EEG." Accessed on January 18, 2018 at https://doi.org/10.1101/125898.

Pattakos, A. (2010) *Prisoners of Our Thoughts: Victor Frankl's Principles for Discovering Meaning in Life and Work*, 2nd edn. San Francisco, CA: Berrett-Koehler Publishers.

Pearson, N., Prosko, S., and Sullivan, M. (eds) (2019) *Yoga and Science in Pain Care: Treating the Person in Pain.* London: Singing Dragon.

Rabey, M. (2017) "A misty, multidimensional crystal ball." *BodyinMind.org.* Accessed on January 18, 2018 at www.bodyinmind.org/low-back-pain-prognosis.

Ray, R. (2000) *Indestructible Truth: The Living Spirituality of Tibetan Buddhism.* Boston, MA: Shambhala.

Robbins, T. and Mallouk, P. (2017) *Unshakeable.* New York: Simon & Schuster.

Rohr, R. (2011) *Falling Upward: A Spirituality for the Two Halves of Life.* Cincinnati, OH: Franciscan Media.

Rohr, R. (2013) *Yes, And…* Cincinnati, OH: Franciscan Media.

Rohr, R. (2017) "Living in Deep Time." Accessed on January 18, 2018 at https://onbeing.org/programs/richard-rohr-living-in-deep-time-apr2017.

Rosenberg, M. B. (2005) "Feelings inventory." Accessed January 23, 2018 at https://www.cnvc.org/Training/feelings-inventory.

Salzberg, S. (2017) "How to Train Your Brain to See Beyond Us Versus Them." Accessed on January 18, 2018 at https://onbeing.org/blog/sharon-salzberg-how-to-train-your-brain-to-see-beyond-us-versus-them.

Scharmer, O. C. (2007) *Theory U: Leading from the Future as It Emerges.* Cambridge, MA: Sol.

Schnäbele, V. (2010) *Yoga in Modern Society.* Hamburg, Germany: Verlag Dr. Kovac.

Senge, P. M., Scharmer, C. O., Jaworksi, J., and Flowers, B. S. (2004) *Presence: Human Purpose and the Field of the Future.* New York: Doubleday.

Siegel, A. and Etzkorn, I. (2013) *Simplicity: Conquering the Crisis of Complexity.* New York: Hachette.

Siegel, D. J. (2017) *Mind: A Journey to the Heart of Being Human.* London: W. W. Norton.

Singleton, M. (2010) *Yoga Body: The Origins of Modern Postural Practice.* New York: Oxford University Press.

Sternberg, R. (1998) "A balance theory of wisdom." *Review of General Psychology 2*, 4, 347–365.

Sullivan, M. B., Moonaz, S., Weber, K., Taylor, J. N., and Schmalzl, L. (2017) "Towards an explanatory framework for yoga therapy informed by philosophical and ethical perspectives." Alternative Therapies in Health and Medicine, Nov 14, pii: AT5717. PMID: 29135457. [Epub ahead of print]

Tagore, R. "The Great Indian Poet and Philosopher Tagore on Truth, Human Nature, and the Interdependence of Existence." Accessed on January 18, 2018 at www.brainpickings. org/2017/03/07/tagore-mans-universe.

Taylor, J. (2008) "End-of-life yoga therapy: Exploring life and death." *International Journal of Yoga Therapy 18*, 97–103.

Taylor, M. J. (2004) "Risk management: Conscious ahimsa." *International Journal of Yoga Therapy 14*, 87–92.

Taylor, M. J. (2006) "Harvesting the full potential of group yoga therapy classes." *International Journal of Yoga Therapy 16*, 33–37.

Taylor, M. J. (2007a) "A fork in the road: "Doing to" or "being with"?" *International Journal of Yoga Therapy 17*, 5–6.

Taylor, M. J. (2007b) "What is yoga therapy? An IAYT definition." *Yoga Therapy in Practice*, 3.

Taylor, M. J. (2015a) "Organizational Yoga Therapy: The Unfoldment of Institutional Yogamind in the World." In *Yoga Therapy: Theory and Practice.* New York: Routledge.

Taylor, M. J. (ed.) (2015b) *Fostering Creativity in Rehabilitation.* New York: Nova Publishing.

Taylor, M. J. and McCall, T (2017) "Implementation of yoga therapy into U.S. healthcare systems." *International Journal of Yoga Therapy 27*, 115–119.

Thompson, E. and Stapleton, M. (2009) "Making sense of sense-making: Reflections on enactive and extended mind theories." *Topoi 28*, 23.

Van de Velde, D., Eijkelkamp, A., Peersman, W., and De Vriendt, P. (2016) "How competent are healthcare professionals in working according to a bio-psycho-social model in healthcare?" *PLOS ONE.* Accessed on January 18, 2018 at http://journals.plos.org/plosone/article?id=10.1371/journal.pone.0164018.

Walsh, R. (2011) "Lifestyle and mental health." *American Psychologist 66*, 7, 579–592.

Walsh, R. (2015) "What is wisdom? Cross-cultural and cross-disciplinary syntheses." *Review of General Psychology 19*, 278–293.

Walsh, R. and Shapiro, S. (2006) "The meeting of meditative disciplines and Western psychology: A mutually enriching dialogue." *American Psychologist 61*, 3, 227–239.

Wolf, C. (2015) "In pain? Try this mindfulness exercise." Accessed January 23, 2018 at https://www.mindful.org/in-pain-try-this-mindfulness-exercise.

Zeidan, F. and Vago, D. (2016) "Mindfulness meditation-based pain relief: A mechanistic account." *Annals of the New York Academy of Sciences 1373*, 1, 114–127.

Zeidan, F., Emerson, N. M., Farris, S. R., Ray, J. N., *et al.* (2015) "Mindfulness meditation-based pain relief employs different neural mechanisms than placebo and sham mindfulness meditation-induced analgesia." *Journal of Neuroscience 35*, 15307–15325.

Subject Index

Author Index

Dr. Matthew J. Taylor, PT, PhD, C-IAYT, leads training programs and creates resources to incorporate smart, safe yoga for the larger yoga community. His leadership in the field of yoga safety and science has made him an expert in chronic pain as well as professional network building for referrals. He is an acknowledged international expert, as well as past-president of the International Association of Yoga Therapists. He continues to serve on their scientific journal's editorial board and as a consultant on their annual Symposium of Yoga Therapy and Research. His Scottsdale, AZ rehabilitation clinic was one of the first clinics ever to be yoga-based. His expertise in clinical application, business development and creativity are all shared in this book. *Yoga Therapy as a Creative Response to Pain* fosters intelligent, creative and tested sources of information and tools for yoga teachers, yoga therapists, and conventional medical professionals who want to incorporate yoga principles into their practices and studios. Personally, he can attribute yoga to both changing his life and easing his chronic back pain. He will guide you through the resources and skills necessary to exceed your goals for supporting your students with chronic pain.